MW01039768

When I was first training to become a heart surgeon, I would look at the heart in awe, because it has this mythical component; [it's regarded as] where the soul is harboured," …"But it changes from being this mythical portion of the body and soul to being a muscle and an anatomic problem that you have to solve.
Heart Surgeon Glen Van Arsdell, Toronto Star

Everyone who is born holds dual citizenship, in the kingdom of the well and in the kingdom of the sick. Although we all prefer to use only the good passport, sooner or later each of us is obliged, at least for a spell, to identify ourselves as citizens of that other place.
Susan Sontag, Author
Cover image: Richard Schwindt and Griffin Metza

Table of Contents

Principles for moving forward

1. You are more than your diagnosis.

Congenital Heart Disease (CHD) or not, we are whole human beings. We have loves, losses, activities, work, education and our human connections. And while this disease can be absorbing, terrifying or debilitating our participation in the world around us keeps us strong.

2. Gather your supports around you

You will needs supports in order to survive. Isolation is a risk factor for ill health. This starts with family, friends and loved ones. It may also include others with CHD, health care providers and anyone else out there who adds to your life in any substantive way.

3. Exercise agency (healthy influence) on your medical care

You cannot control your health, others or the medical system, nor should you. But you can be an informed and engaged patient or stakeholder. This is crucial to optimizing your care and ensuring that you are at the centre of decisions made about you. You may not be an expert on CHD but you can be the leading expert on (your name, or your child's name).

4. Care for the rest of your body

Basic self-care is important for anyone but more so for CHD patients. Are you eating well? Sleeping? Exercising? Staying hydrated? All of these things are important; your body is much more than your heart

5. Manage your emotions, particularly anxiety

The constellation of emotions effecting those with CHD includes the positive (joy, gratitude, love) and those that trouble us, (fear, guilt, anger and sadness). Fear and anxiety can limit us and prevent us from engaging in the world.

Introduction

Much of what is accomplished in the world is accomplished by people who aren't feeling very good today.
Eleanor Roosevelt

What is congenital heart disease? To begin with, it is complicated. Present from birth, it embraces all the weird and bad things that can happen to what should be a fairly straightforward organ: a muscle with four chambers. Numerous things can go wrong, some of which are inconvenient and others life threatening.

My father had congenital heart disease diagnosed late in life. I have CHD that was life threatening at the time of my birth. And my grandson, Griffin, has a more serious version than me. My father had heart surgery in his seventies. I had surgery at ages two and 45, and my grandson was operated on three times before he was two.

Without minimizing the effect of CHD, it has been both a curse and a blessing in my life. In a quiet room you can hear my mechanical mitral valve tick. I preach the merits of home based INR (blood coagulation) testing. I call my doctors plumbers and electricians and have watched at least one of them start young and grow old. I have a hilarious relationship with anxiety and can do the one hour mile.

A marvel of adjustment and adaptation, I have had a full life as a husband, father, grandfather, therapist and writer. I have spent the last thirty five years helping those who struggle with their emotions and managing my own. I have worked with both children and adults through illness, loss, love, survival and tragedy. And now I want to turn my attention to children, teens and adults who struggle with the emotional aftermath of CHD.

I'm focusing on helping people who struggle with the emotional turbulence resulting from a CHD diagnosis; adults, children, siblings, partners. The focus on everyone in the story reflects one piece of evidence based *knowledge* and one *principle*.

Knowledge: Children evolve into adults surrounded by family, friends and other social connections.

Principle: My deepest and earliest training is as a systemic family therapist. That means that I look at the ecology of family and community systems to understand individuals. In addition I watch for my client's success in navigating their own milestones and those in the developmental cycle of their family.

Julie and Tony were in their mid-thirties and desperately wanted to start a family. They were frightened that any child born to them would inherit Julie's CHD and Tony's parents insisted that it would be irresponsible for them to have a child given Julie's illness. In counselling it was agreed that in order to move forward (in their family life cycle) they would need to make their own decision about children. They decided to seek genetic counselling in order to make an informed choice.

This book is not going to spend much time on medical questions (where I am not qualified), but more on our emotional responses to visits, procedures, surgery, medication and, most importantly, how we live our lives.

Although I will touch on my own experience as a CHD patient and that of my grandson, Griffin, this book is more about providing you with tools, ideas and the philosophical basis to move forward and live a fulfilling life, no matter what the state of yours or your loved ones health.

People with CHD and those who care for them spend a lot of time managing fear, considering lifestyle choices, coping with the medical system, finances, body image and their larger relationship with the world. While there is material out there on coping with CHD it tends to be filtered through sincere helpers and the medical system. This is good but the *Emotional Recovery from…* series is rooted in day to day practical engagement with the world. As human beings we work, relate, have sex, play, drink beer with the gals, travel to Europe, and sign up for white water rafting.

As human beings we are wired to balance need (eat, sleep, mate) with caution (there could be a sabre tooth tiger behind that rock). When we get excited, frightened or active, our body has a multitude of emotional and physical responses; our respiration changes, muscles tense up, temperature changes and, oh yes, our heart responds. That last part can be dodgy for CHD patients because our hearts don't always respond or they respond in strange ways (too fast, too slow, out of sync). This has the chicken/egg response that often drives people with perfectly good hearts to cardiologists after a panic attack.

It is often appropriate to rule out heart disease if you suffer from panic but panic can make your heart misbehave and your heart misbehaving can – that's right – create panic. While our heart sped up historically when a tiger appeared our heart can speed up now when our unconscious mind thinks: *"That tiger must be around here somewhere."*

This book will identify and normalize some of the things that you are feeling and provide tools that you can use to manage the emotions and particular circumstances faced by CHD patients and their families. I will be drawing from my own and my family's experience, thirty five years as a practising therapist and the literature that I find helpful. That said, the thoughts expressed are my own.

I like to use case examples. All the case examples in this book are either fabricated or changed to the point of being unrecognizable.

Finally, to a great extent, I cope with humour. Flip, silly, snarky or dark; I'm cool with it all. It sneaks into my writing whether I try to suppress it or not. Bear in mind that Mister Anxiety (more on him later) has a few mortal enemies and first among them is laughter.

This book in the end celebrates the life we create for ourselves.

On emotions

Never apologize for showing feeling. When you do so, you apologize for the truth.
Benjamin Disraeli

Honeybees pollinate plants and bats eat mosquitos. They are our friends and yet when directly encountered we step back.

If we receive an injury on our body it may turn red, bruise, swell and hurt. This is unpleasant but these symptoms serve a purpose in healing.

Likewise with our emotions. So many of my clients fear them in themselves or others. Emotions are innate within us and exist for a reason. While most of us are fine when we experience joy, laughter, hope and love, we may go into denial when we experience anger, fear, sadness, and guilt. Or we may turn away when we witness these emotions in others.

Accept what you feel and don't take what others feel too personally.

You are more than
your diagnosis

I didn't expect to recover from my second operation but since I did, I consider that I'm living on borrowed time. Every day that dawns is a gift to me and I take it in that way. I accept it gratefully without looking beyond it. I completely forget my physical suffering and all the unpleasantness of my present condition and I think only of the joy of seeing the sun rise once more and of being able to work a little bit,
even under difficult conditions.
Henri Matisse

We all have reason to be here. And most of us have obstacles to achieving happiness and our life's goals. People struggle with, loss, terrible work stress, marital and family issues, physical illness, mental illness, trauma from accidents and abuse. It is rare – and frankly undesirable - to go through life unscathed by adversity. As much as we don't wish it on ourselves or others, it does shape us. I see some people broken and embitterdes by their experiences but more often I see people triumph.

There are four practical problems that CHD can create in your life, whether you or someone you love has it.

1. Much of your time is consumed by appointments, care, hospitalization, and recovery.

2. Your energy, activity and wellbeing
    are challenged by the limits of your
    cardiovascular system.

3. Depending on where you live, your work,
    insurance coverage etc. your medical costs
    and cost in time away from work may cause
    considerable strain.

4. You are unclear about the extent of the
    first three.

Tim's surgery was scheduled for early fall, pending the surgeon's schedule. The surgery was hopefully going to help but there would be a period of recovery. He did not know if he would available, or even up to going back to college in January.

Supports may be limited. All of these obstacles are real and coloured by the overt or covert fear of mortality. What if we die? What if our child dies? These thoughts and their emotional associations can take us right to a black and despairing place. Although few fields have progressed as much as the treatment of CHD, much of it remains invasive, often involving surgical solutions and powerful medication.

And yet, we are to a certain extent, designed to fear the worst. And there is nothing that screams *"game over, man"* like, say, the inside of a Cath lab (aka a heart catheterization lab). And the whole procedure might start with someone helpfully telling you how many people actually die during the procedure. The numbers might be quite small but the loss aversion mechanisms of our psych go right to the number of people who succumb *in this very location* as opposed to the large majority for whom the procedure produces valuable and life-saving information. Our fear in this situation might be based on something a cognitive behavioral therapist would call a cognitive distortion.

We are here to live our lives and the choices available for living those lives while not limitless are abundant. It is probably better that having made sure that we can't do something (be sure about that; you might be wrong) we move towards and celebrate the things that we can. As human beings we generally are going to want to pursue stimulating activities, work at something where we can make a living and feel fulfilled, partner up, have sex, have children, and live a long life. All of us have to understand that we need to make those opportunities for ourselves and sometimes they will involve risk.

Christos was sure he would never have sex and when the opportunity arose he was terrified. No woman would desire a guy with scars across his chest. He was astounded that his girlfriend didn't even seem to notice.

Risk aversion can be even worse if it's not you taking the risk.

When Kyle went to cub camp for the first time he was just eight. His parents were terrified. What if he got sick? What if he couldn't handle the hikes? Kyle came back bedraggled with half his gear missing. He told them that it was the best weekend he had ever spent.

This is the philosophic core of the book. No matter the obstacles in our path we need to go forward.

"Courage is not the absence of fear, but rather the judgement that something else is more important than fear."

Ambrose Redmoon

Gather your
supports around you

A true friend encourages us, comforts us, supports us like a big easy chair, offering us a safe refuge from the world.
H. Jackson Brown, Jr.

When trouble comes, it's your family that supports you.
Guy Lafleur

People in the medical and health world look at risk factors. So do those who provide therapy or emotional care. Understanding risk factors tell us much about the challenges ahead and how they will be met.

Evan had excellent medical care but was forgetful of his medication, smoked like a chimney and rarely ventured off the couch.

See any risk factors there? Now let's add something that I consider the primary emotional risk, which at the same time is recognized as a physical risk as well.

Evan had few friends, nor did he have a job and coworkers. Following a series of disputes with his father he had stepped back from his family.

I consider Evan's risk to be considerable. Human beings are social animals. Like llamas and marmots we are gregarious and wither in isolation. We need the strokes - physical and emotional - that come with having people around. Even bad or conflictual relationships can meet these needs to a certain extent. In communities that shun or banish a person, the banished individual often dies.

On a practical level people who love us want us to take care of ourselves. They give us grief if we don't take our meds, take us to appointments and drive us home from procedures. They can be impatient with our sickness which contributes to our motivation to get well.

They make us do things we don't feel like doing and are close by if there is a crisis. Since we love them we want to get better. In my practice the number one reason despairing people tell me why they don't kill themselves is: *"I wouldn't do that to my family"*.

If we have kids or dependents we have increased motivation to get better. If we have co-workers, clients, patients, students or customers, we don't want to let them down.

> *Really sick people don't make up frivolous excuses to miss work. I have seen cancer patients bring a bucket to put beside their desk in case they had to throw up.*
> *Hospital Staff heath nurse in Sioux Lookout*

I had a man working for me as a therapist for four years in Sioux Lookout. He had type one diabetes and he didn't take a sick day in the four years. Once there was a blizzard, and the highway was closed. He lived ten miles out of town. I spoke to him over the phone and laughed: *"Got you this time bud, you have a day off whether you like it or not."*

Ninety minutes later I was shocked to find him at his desk.

"Did they open the highway?"

"No, I skied across the lake."

It is other people that get us through. That said, relationships and social connections need to be nurtured. We need two skills: helping others, and reaching out for help when we need it. People tend to be much better at one than the other.

Abdul: I help people all the time and now that I need support no one comes around. People will really let you down.

I would suggest that Abdul take another approach.

Abdul: When I got sick I knew I couldn't do it alone. I picked up the phone and called a few people. Not everyone was able to help but a buddy did my lawn this week and another friend did some cooking. The little things make a difference.

Also, in the modern era there are groups online; parents, patients and others who support each other and share experiences. The world feels different when you are part of a group. You know who understands the experience of raising a child with heart problems? Another parent of a child with heart problems.

Other supports:

Professional supports

As CHD patients we tend to think of medical staff as our professional supports but there are many others if we expand our thinking a little. Here are a few:

Professional Emotional Healers

By professional healer I mean a person with some form of advanced education in a helping field who adheres to recognized standards of practise and ethical guidelines. (Usually a professional college or association). It does not mean that other healers lack skill or ethics; it is just that members of a professional association are accountable to clear expectations as to how they conduct their work.

Although many professionals will have some knowledge of the issues around CHD, most will not understand the psychological symptoms. Help them. A good therapist is always open to your input.

Note that there are some professional emotional helpers, particularly around teaching hospitals, with special knowledge and understanding of Congenital Heart Disease.

A *Psychologist* normally has a doctorate in Psychology and is registered as a Psychologist in his/her jurisdiction. Some specialize in psychological testing and research but many are excellent therapists. They are on the expensive side but partially covered with many insurance plans.

Psychiatrists are what many people inexperienced with therapy think of first. As medical specialists, they are responsible for medical units and psychiatric programs and many specialize in diagnosis, serious mental illness and medication. It can be quite difficult to find one without a referral, though when you do they are often covered under insurance or provincial health plans. It is more difficult to find one who specializes in psychotherapy.

Many *Social Workers* have extensive training in psychotherapy and do it every day. They are cheaper than psychologists, more available, and who you are likely to run into if you are seen in a social agency or a workplace Employee Assistance Program. More and more they are covered under insurance and extended health plans.

Historically the term *Psychotherapist* had no precise meaning and could be used by anyone. In Ontario that has changed and it has a precise meaning now, given to people who are members of the Ontario College of Psychotherapy. There are a number of people who might practice psychotherapy, potentially including *nurses*, people with *masters' level training in psychology*, *occupational therapists* and *clergy*. Remember that doing psychotherapy or counseling well is a challenging career-long commitment, not a sidebar or hobby. Also bear in mind that the difference between counseling and psychotherapy to a great extent is in the eye of the beholder. I would argue that psychotherapy is a deeper process but the important question for you to ask is what it means to the person you go to for help.

While many grumble about *Family Physicians* doing therapy the truth is that much of their day is occupied doing therapy on the fly. And they have the added advantage of knowing the medical issues and prescription rights. There are some who do specialize in delivering therapy. Many psychological issues arise from physiological illness.

Alternate or Holistic Healers

> *(I've)....started practicing yoga. I started learning some hands-on healing stuff. And I found really good chiropractors, really good massage therapists, and what I found is I've been able to actually peel off layers of trauma on my body and actually move better now than I did.*
> *Ricky Williams*

I'm referring here of people like *acupuncturists, massage therapists, chiropractors, naturopaths* and others who practice forms of healing that directly involve your body.

If you open your mind you may find that there are people out there who can provide support through *Reikki, Acupuncture, hypnotherapy, Yoga, Tai Chi, Neurofeedback, Bodytalk* and a host of other approaches to mind and body. Again, these approaches typically cost money but if you check around with your friends you may find out who is out there and recommended.

Many of these approaches nurture your spirit as well as your body. Some practitioners may be special individuals who seem to have gifts of insight and touch. It is worth finding out who they are.

Even looking at my short list here there are considerable differences in education, outlook and the nature of the work. Any of the above for example might treat anxiety, which has many physical manifestations. If they are making physical interventions you will want to ensure that they do not negatively impact your medical care (e.g. herbal treatments that interact with heart medication).

Spiritual Healers

> *Science is not only compatible with spirituality; it is a profound source of spirituality. When we recognize our place in an immensity of light-years and in the passage of ages, when we grasp the intricacy, beauty, and subtlety of life, then that soaring feeling, that sense of elation and humility combined, is surely spiritual. So are our emotions in the presence of great art or music or literature, or acts of exemplary selfless courage such as those of Mahatma Gandhi or Martin Luther King, Jr. The notion that science and spirituality are somehow mutually exclusive does a disservice to both.*
> *Carl Sagan*

We are mind, body and spirit. You may not adhere to any particular faith or you may even be a principled atheist.

Either way, there is another dimension of your life that needs to be acknowledged and brought into the healing constellation.

Historically spiritual healers have much emotional healing, regardless of their group, sect or denomination. While this category of healer embraces some charlatans the spiritual dimension of healing is often ignored by other professionals. There are traditions of healing in all the major religions. Christians have prayer services, Islamic people consult with the Koran, Wiccans cast healing spells and First Nations people may use sweat lodges and shaking tents. Principled atheists draw on larger principles of how we coexist with our fellow human beings.

Financial Healers

From the spiritual to the pragmatic, we run across the issue of money. Many of the causes of anxiety can lead to financial setbacks. Often people with severe anxiety, illness or abuse issues are temporarily unable to work. These are real concerns; most of us need to work and maintain an income. Knowing that you may have trouble with the rent or the kid's school expenses will do nothing to reduce anxiety. Having a carefully thought out financial plan that identifies your net worth, assets and debts will help you make decisions in an informed manner. I am always struck by bankers I know or counsel who tell me the most satisfying part of their job is helping out people who are struggling. Many care deeply about what they do. Consider making a financial advisor part of your recovery team.

Social Agencies

By social agencies I mean not-for-profit organizations funded through charitable or government sources. These include hospital departments, community mental health programs, children's mental health centres, and a wide range of organizations that address mental health, addictions, and family and life issues. Approach them as a polite but assertive consumer. Bringing your understanding of CHD to the table will help.

Employee Assistance Programs (EAP)

Much of the counseling done in Canada and the United States is provided by EAP providers. These are private organizations that are hired by the company you work for to provide counseling services. The services are generally confidential and the records inaccessible to your employer. Also, the services are normally short term with a component to help with crisis situations. The quality of EAP counselors is usually good to excellent.

Vocational Counsellors

Some people with CHD underachieve. There may be someone in your community who can help you make the most of your skills and strengths.

Exercise agency
(healthy influence)
on your medical care

It will never rain roses: when we want to have more roses, we must plant more roses.
George Eliot

Don't wait for your ship to come in, swim out to it.
Cathy Hopkins

I had a friend – an engineer and one of the brightest people I knew – tell me that he had started on the anticoagulant, Warfarin. I asked him what his INR was. He replied: *"What's that?"*

(Note that all medications have an official or scientific name and a brand name. The brand name may vary from country to country. For example, Coumadin is a brand name for Warfarin. It is also known as Marevan in the UK.)

INR stands for International Normalized Ratio but in the end it is a number that indicates the ability and speed of blood coagulation. This number is discerned through a blood test. I explained it to him and encouraged him to find out from his doctor the numbers that were right for him. I try to keep mine, for example, between 3 and 3.5.

That is actually a high number but recommended by my cardiologist based on my mechanical mitral valve and history of having a stroke. Everyone is different.

This points to a different concern. My friend had only recently learned of his diagnosis and he was scared. Understanding the subtleties of Warfarin would confront him with the frightening emotional reality of heart disease.

Denial can be a judgemental term. Better to think of it as a stage in Elizabeth Kubler Ross's stages of grief, (*denial, anger, bargaining, depression, acceptance*). However, people can get stuck there.

How many times has the doctor's office staff asked you to bring your meds in a bag to her office? I find that a little infantilizing but I do understand it. Many of my own clients on anti-depressant or sleeping medication have no idea what they are taking. One of them produced a bag of her meds the other day and I found it helpful to see them directly and discuss them with her.

Accepting your situation is one way we can interact intelligently with the medical system and ensure that we are doing everything outside of medical contacts to keep ourselves healthy and well. To illustrate this point I want to compare the stories of Liang and Sarah.

Sarah is 55 and a smoker. She has been healthy all her life but focused on a stressful career. Last week she had a terrifying experience that began with excruciating chest pains. She didn't go to the hospital right away because she was trying to complete a work project. However, after 24 hours her husband had enough and called an ambulance himself. With the paramedics he persuaded her to get help. In hospital she received an angiogram and was quickly scheduled for surgery. Following the surgery the medical staff presented her with some stark choices. She needed to examine her stress levels, change her diet and begin an exercise program. She had new medication to take and had to quit smoking. The hospital was offering a consult with a dietician, a heart attack recovery group and referral to a smoke ending program.

Now, let's look at another case:

Liang, 50, was diagnosed with type one diabetes as a young boy. He measured his blood sugar, monitored his blood sugar readings and injected himself with insulin throughout his childhood and youth. He attended the diabetes clinic and went to diabetes camp. Still, diabetes is always challenging and comes with an increased risk of heart disease. That said, when the chest pains came Liang turned to his wife and said, "We have to get to the hospital right now." Liang is an imperfect man and was frightened by the heart attack but he is bearing up well and working with the hospital staff to plan for his release and new reality.

There are some obvious differences between Sarah and Liang. She has been healthy her whole life. This came as a visceral shock and the thirty year reality of stressful work temporarily trumped her need for immediate medical care. She was unfamiliar with the medical system and scared to feel so vulnerable.

Liang on the other hand has been in training for this moment since he was a child. He is as upset as Sarah but familiar with the medical system and focused self-care. He is able to immediately exercise agency which puts him ahead of Sarah both in terms of making the most of the care available and his emotional recovery.

So where does that put CHD patients? We have had health challenges since the beginning though our personal experiences are quite varied, depending on the seriousness of the disease and the amount of intervention needed.

We may have never been the "invincible" teenager who thought nothing could happen to them. On the other hand we might have had CHD with few symptoms or interventions needed that flared up at some point and required procedures or surgery. That can come as a shock.

What strikes me about both those stories is that Liang's lifetime of needing to care for his own health has provided him with great agency or ability to influence (not control) his health for the better. There are many successful type one diabetic people who would go downhill fast without excellent self-care. Mr. Perfect Health over there can get away with a bad diet and sedentary lifestyle (at least for now), but some of us don't have that choice.

Here is another example. I have a Coaguchek monitor to measure my INR. It is quick, effective, evidence based and can go along with me when I travel. It saves me trips downtown to the blood technician who may or may not find my vein with the first poke. So why are they not in common use? Warfarin/Coumadin is commonly used, not just by heart patients but by many others who might be prone to clots.

And yet I have run into headwinds promoting this to medical practitioners who don't think their patients are up to the simple finger prick test, let alone adjusting their medication. Hence my admonition: "*I am not dumber than a diabetic,*" who does this every day.

Self-measurement is not for everyone but it is one example of the many ways that people help themselves stay well. My point is that pro-active care is as important for your emotional health as it is for your physical health.

Although I am primarily a therapist you cannot have a career in social work without developing case management skills. And my most important case is me. My daughter, Elisa, is Griffin's case manager. Every case needs one.

Interacting with medical staff and system

Greg and Anne met with the cardiologist about their two year old son, Nathan. After the meeting they felt confused and rushed. There were questions they had not asked and things the cardiologist had said that seemed to contradict what another doctor told them. On the drive home Greg said, "I'm sick of this crap. They only care about getting you in one door and out the other." Anne, who had been through so many of these meetings, started to cry. Nathan, sitting in the back seat, felt scared and started to cry himself.

The medical system is large, complex and populated by human beings with all their strengths and flaws. Much of what happens seems beyond our understanding and mistakes get made. The medical staff may be highly skilled and committed but we are dealing with our lives or the lives of our children and therefore have a different and more intense emotional engagement.

It is easy to become overwhelmed when talking to medical staff. We may not understand their specific role and much of what they say. We can devolve to an infantilized or vulnerable state where we hear things selectively.

When Corey's cardiologist discussed the risks in the coming procedure he noted a one percent risk of serious complication. Corey felt himself stiffen. He was unaware that the doctor had just told him that in ninety-nine percent of cases there were no serious complications.

Medical staff are usually acutely aware of what they say. However, their statements can sound contrived and moreover; we often go into a bit of trance state. Any hesitation or error in tone can cause fear and rumination in the patient. I am a hypnotherapist and have taken a courses in medical hypnotherapy. Did you know there was such a thing? It sometimes involves people who provide hypnotic suggestions and intervention in an ER or in crisis situations.

So, does emergency hypnotherapy involve long inductions, counting down or waving a watch? *No, the patients, through fear or trauma, are already in a trance state.* What we know is that in a trance the unconscious mind comes forward. The unconscious mind is suggestible and literal. This means that the doctor has to frame her statement so that the messaging is received accurately and is put into proper perspective by the patient or his/her parents.

A staff member was caught in traffic and would not arrive at the hospital in time for rounds. Asked by a doctor about his attendance, the nurse said, "He's not going to make it." She was standing outside Edward's room when she said this and shortly after discovered Edward hyperventilating.

Ellen was a successful lawyer. She walked into the hospital for her heart catheterization in a business suit. Before two hours had passed she had no underwear, her groin was shaved, blood was drawn, intravenous inserted and she lay on the bed in a gown that opened at the back. She felt like she had been reduced to the state of a terrified and helpless child.

We can feel like a piece of meat. In the medical system there are tasks that need to be done to screen patients and ensure that they are ready for a procedure or meeting. The doctor needs specific data to make her decision. Most high end medical facilities have both the blessing and curse of volume. This is important to understand.

The blessing of volume is that it produces a critical mass of information for research and evaluation of best practises. In addition, the more cases seen by any individual in the system the greater their personal feeling for and understanding of the phenomenon.

It is better to have the guy who has performed the procedure a thousand times rather than a hundred times.

In my job as a therapist I sometimes point to the right side of my head and say that "this side cares about the people I see." I then point to the left and say, "This side calculates data and directs the next step. I need both sides of my brain to do therapy."

One downside of high volume is that it feels impersonal. On the assembly line of patients you are next up. Unlike me, doctors, nurses and technicians have to overbalance towards that calculating left side. This is, in the end, a good thing.

For a doctor seeing many patients the data allows them to make fact based decisions. This does not mean they should abandon compassion and the need to factor in a patient's emotional state, but it helps to understand their mindset.

I approach fearful things in the medical system much the same way I approach flying. When I flew often in small planes, I made a study of how planes used the shape of their wings to get off the ground, the sounds they made, the risks associated with turbulence and reasonable safety measures. For example, we worry about crashing but you are much more likely to get bumped on the noggin if the pilot puts the seatbelt light on as you fly into turbulence and you don't comply.

My approach rarely eliminates fear but it does help me manage it.

Being in that calculating side of the head puts us in the game and allows us to manage our emotions and have *agency* at the same time. If the doctor or nurse leaves and you still have questions, ask someone else. Yes, you have a right to have your questions answered but polite perseverance is the most effective strategy to making this happen.

Mistakes will be made. This will not be the result of callous medical staff or underfunding or human stupidity, but because of the inevitable flaws in a complex and high volume environment. Everyone involved, the medical staff, and you, has a responsibility to catch the mistakes.

Shareema noticed that her medication wasn't given at bedtime. The doctor came in and she reminded him. He didn't apologise or seem to notice. She again reminded the nurse. Shortly after the medication arrived.

If Shareema hadn't spoken up maybe someone would have remembered the medication. Maybe she would have missed one dose and it would have not been a big deal. Maybe someone would have come in and explained why they weren't giving that medication that night. However, something that could have been a problem was greatly simplified because she sought out an explanation.

In the real world medical personnel don't like to lose face or admit errors. What they like to do is catch mistakes before they start, correct them and move forward.

There is no point in being affronted, shocked or cynical about the medical system. We all know there are flaws. In the face of genuine neglect or malpractice there may be other steps that need to be taken but the majority of medical screw ups are going to be the outcome of errors by busy human beings. Do your bit to ensure this does not happen to you or someone you love.

If you believe that underfunding, wait lists etc. are an issue in your program you may choose to get together with others who share the same concern or make your voice heard on a political level. Advocating on behalf of CHD patients is itself a form of emotional healing.

Care for the rest of your body

I do yoga, I do Bikram and I run,
and I eat really healthy.
Lady Gaga

A few years back I attended training with the Canadian Society for Clinical Hypnosis taught by Dr. Max Shapiro, a leading hypnotherapist and psychologist from Yale University. It was a great two days but I was struck by his insistence on asking each client four questions on their physical self-care:

Are you sleeping?

Are you eating properly?

Are you getting exercise?

Are you staying hydrated?

He was clear that without self-care the techniques in his arsenal would be useless.

The need to take care of ourselves under stress is obvious and yet, now that I have incorporated these questions into my practise I see how often they are neglected. They represent the low hanging fruit of healing. I see anxious people in a high state of physiological arousal (stressed). Self-care activities should de-stimulate as well as maintain wellness.

Of all these activities sleep is perhaps the most problematic. Most people claim to understand the basics of sleep hygiene, even if it is not practised. At the core is your need to de-stimulate in the hours before bed and use the bedroom only for sleep and sex. So no workout tapes, spicy vindaloo, espresso, Metallica tapes or Vin Diesel movies at the end of the night and especially not in the bedroom. Leave your Blackberry in the den.

This much is obvious. So obvious in fact that people who try all this stuff, throw in some sleep medication, and still don't sleep, get freaked out. They are convinced that they are going to turn into walking zombies. It helps to get your head to equate rest and sleep and learn to enjoy the quiet hours. You can reframe your state: why not lay there, rest and let your brain off the hook for a bit. You might try meditation, self-hypnosis, or just lying there doing nothing.

This is critical because if you start to become anxious about your sleep you are going to have an adrenal response where your unconscious mind goes into crisis mode. Suddenly your mind and body are on full alert and prepared for action.

If you have CHD you may also have to factor in a rapid or erratic heartbeat, or perhaps shortness of breath. You may have to seek medical solutions to these issues but in the meantime you could consider integrating them into your sleep. Here is a simple hypnosis technique for sleep. Note the way the environment with its sounds and sensations are incorporated into the messaging. In the end you have to reinterpret the distractions as sleep aids.

Self-hypnosis (a simple sleep technique)

Become aware of your breathing; try counting your breaths up to ten and down again. Or reversing "breathe in, breathe out" to "breathe out, breathe in".....

Be aware of the support the bed is giving your body and the pillow your head...

Put your mind in each toe, then each foot then your ankle and work your way up....

Give yourself the explicit message that all sounds inside and outside the bedroom are helping you to rest and the only sound that matters is the sound of your inner voice....

Imagine your favourite kind of flower; in your mind's eye, look at it, smell it, touch it and imagine the sound a breeze might make as it brushes by. Now change the flower and see how it looks in another colour or with other flowers....

Introduce a mantra or phrase; it should be positive because the message will be going directly to your unconscious mind (e.g. "God's Peace" or "Quiet Rest")

Our bodies need sleep and they need exercise. Our bodies are built to move. This is one area where you want to be clear with your medical provider. Find out exactly how much exercise you can tolerate and go for it. You may find that you can do more than you assumed.

The only restriction ever put on me involved common sense and a restriction against ice hockey when I was a kid. A couple of years ago my cardiologist suggested I stop lifting heavy weights. Exercise is good for your body and it is also good for your emotional recovery.

In research of treatment for mild to moderate depression and anxiety, exercise has been demonstrated to be as effective as medication and therapy.

That's right. A good walking regime can be as effective as Prozac and Cognitive Behavioral Therapy.

We don't eat normally when we are anxious or stressed. Many of my clients confess to binging on junk food for the salty\sugary\fatty respite. Some lose weight. When I see diabetics under stress their sugars are all over the map. I am not an expert on nutrition but many experts claim there is a correlation between diet and mood. Check this out and move towards the diet that works for you. Make sure you understand the dietary implications of your meds.

Robert told me in my office that since starting on Warfarin he had stopped eating all vegetables.

I sent Robert back to his doctor after trying to explain that the dosage of his Warfarin had to be adjusted according to the amount of vitamin K rich food he ate and his individual response to the drug. But he was in despair in advance of understanding the facts.

And allow me to state the obvious, *caffeine makes anxiety worse.* Most of us want our coffee in the morning but whether you get it through coffee, cola or chocolate caffeine remains a stimulant drug. Moreover, it has a stimulating effect on your heart, which may not be a great idea.

People get dehydrated and don't know it. According to the Mayo Clinic website:

Water is your body's principal chemical component and makes up about 60 percent of your body weight. Every system in your body depends on water. For example, water flushes toxins out of vital organs, carries nutrients to your cells and provides a moist environment for ear, nose and throat tissues.

It goes on to say that we can become hydrated from both liquid and food sources men need roughly 13 cups of liquid a day and women, nine. In the end it is not far from the eight glasses of water we have been hearing about for years.

Again, there may be implications and/or restrictions for CHD patients, particularly those with heart failure or those taking diuretics.

A word on evidence based care

A wise man proportions his belief to the evidence.
David Hume

I wanted to make a comment on the concept of evidence based care. There is always research underway and new results are always being published. Part of the art of medicine is knowing and evaluating research results and adjusting practice accordingly. Complicating this is the fact that research results sometimes contradict other research results, or may use questionable methodology.

The results are often debated and occasionally long standing truths are overturned. That said, most research is responsible and most medical organizations do their best to ensure that evidence in incorporated into practice. Occasional travesties of research (e.g. the myth that vaccination is linked to autism), are discredited.

It is worth noting that approaches to psychotherapy and emotional healing should also be evidence based but there is a debate in the field as to what that means. The classic approach to evidence based practice suggested that you could prescribe a specific approach to a specific diagnosis. (e.g. Cognitive Behavioral Therapy for anxiety).

While CBT is very helpful for anxiety, there are other approaches. Taking from the work of researchers Michael Lambert, Scott Miller, Barry Duncan and others, many of us believe that effective change comes from four factors in this order of importance:

1. The cumulative actions of the client in all settings

2. Rapport with therapist

3. The quality of hope

4. The specific approach to therapy (e.g. CBT)

This has some significant implications. The above researchers would note the need for *practice based evidence*; in other words, the continual use of feedback from the client. So let's take a hypothetical example of Julie who is suffering from anxiety.

1. *Julie decided that she didn't want her life controlled by her anxiety. In the same week, she started yoga, met with her family doctor, improved her diet and started with a therapist.*

2. *The therapist was respectful and open. He appeared knowledgeable and was genuinely interested in her opinions and feedback. She shared with him that she had tried CBT before and didn't find it helpful. Based on his skill set she decided to try some hypnotherapy. After a session of hypnotherapy she told him it was relaxing and helpful.*

3. *Julie started to feel more hopeful and optimistic about challenging her anxiety.*

4. *They stuck with hypnosis but in another circumstance they might have used Mindfulness, CBT, or Brief Solution Focused therapy with good results.*

You can see that Julie's means of addressing anxiety embraces much more than a counselling methodology. In the end she has set a comprehensive process in motion to feel better.

Approaches that have been proven in psychological research are great but remember that other approaches might relax you and lift your spirit; the more comprehensive your approach to emotional issues the more likely it is to work. My personal observation of how good therapists approach their own problems is that they "throw the kitchen sink at them."

Manage your emotions, particularly anxiety

> *The mind is powerful, and you have more*
> *control than you think.*
> *Scott D. Lewis,*

Many CHD people are anxious and don't understand or acknowledge it. This can take the form of the controlling or angry person who believes they can externalize their emotions rather than admit: "I'm scared." It can also take the form of the withdrawn person who gradually moves away from social involvement and society at large. Some people can go their entire lives with terrible fear and never show or acknowledge it. Some self-medicate with addictive behaviors.

This is not the way it needs to be; anxiety is treatable. As I tell my clients: "*We have the technology.*" One of the assumptions of this series of books is that emotional recovery is possible and there are many ways to achieve it. This is not fantasy. Most of my clients finish work with me better than they started.

This is not because I am a clinical genius but because they brought the power of *intent* into the office. Their calling for help often coincided with a call to the family doctor, picking up some reading material and development of a personal self-care regimen.

There is a psychology and attitude to managing anxiety. It involves *flowing into the anxiety* and, as strange as this sounds, not taking it too seriously. When I tell my clients that, they are sometimes a little put off.

Richard doesn't take my anxiety seriously? It's destroying my life!

Not to panic (pun intended), but you can mount a vigorous campaign to control and even eliminate anxiety and have some fun along the way. I know that sound contradictory but *Mr. Anxiety* – a concrete metaphor - counts on you taking him seriously. I also understand that anxiety at its worst is a severe illness that requires psychiatric care.

> *I must say a word about fear. It is life's only true opponent. Only fear can defeat life. It is a clever, treacherous adversary, how well I know. It has no decency, respects no law or convention, shows no mercy. It goes for your weakest spot, which it finds with unnerving ease. It begins in your mind, always ... so you must fight hard to express it. You must fight hard to shine the light of words upon it. Because if you don't, if your fear becomes a wordless darkness that you avoid, perhaps even manage to forget, you open yourself to further attacks of fear because you never ruly fought the opponent who defeated you.*
> *Yann Martel, Life of Pi*

Mr. Anxiety showed up when I was counselling a child. I do some of my best work with children because they force me to be clear, simple and straightforward. I take what I learn and use it with adults. In my office I stand up and put my hands over my head and say "grr grr". Mr. Anxiety is an imposing presence but also an imposter. He whispers bad things:

You are going to fail

You can't go on this trip

You can't handle needles

You are too weak to go out

You are sick

You will never feel better

This procedure is going to hurt

The operation is going to fail

You are going to die

Your daughter won't make it

I show myself backing away from Mr. Anxiety, shrinking and withdrawing into a corner. Now I demonstrate how much Mr. Anxiety likes my fear as he grows in strength and ferocity.

Then I show myself responding differently to Mr. Anxiety; darting towards him, shaking hands with him, laughing at him, embracing him. *Now it is Mr. Anxiety shrinking into the corner.*

This illustrates a fundamental concept of addressing anxiety: *flow into anxiety.*

Depression

Dr. Edward Shorter is a psychiatric historian. In his wonderful book *How Everyone Became Depressed: The Rise and Fall of the Nervous Breakdown,* he notes that throughout history a cluster of five symptoms: anxiety, depression, intrusive thoughts, somatic (physical) symptoms and fatigue have been found together and at this stage of our history are usually identified as depression.

He believes that when we identified these symptoms as "nerves" we had a paradigm that rang true for sufferers. He also suggests that calming the body and the mind were and are effective management strategies.

If you have CHD you are going to be more aware of the somatic side than most. Similarly, you may feel fatigued for reasons associated with your illness and perhaps reasons unrelated. I recall one time going to the cardiologist for fatigue and after he had done the tests and evaluation he declared my heart stable. He was getting up to leave when I asked, *"Why am I so tired?"*

He turned on his way out and said: *"Life Stress?"*

Don't judge yourself too harshly for worrying that every symptom is heart related. Adopting a balanced approach to evaluating and caring for your health, having a good sense of your emotional makeup and maybe using some cognitive behavioral therapy for sorting through your thoughts will help you learn to discern emotional from physical symptoms. If you have an embarrassing moment at a medical facility laugh at yourself then laugh it off.

Still as many as one person in five will receive a diagnosis of depression at one time or another. Some who have a deep debilitating illness, and a larger group who still function more or less but under a cloud. Here are some common indicators:

Feelings of sadness

Feelings of hopelessness

Loss of self-confidence

Feeling that life isn't worth living

Lack of energy

Loss of interest in daily activities

Inability to experience pleasure

Restlessness or agitation

Feelings of shame or guilt

Poor concentration or memory

Change in libido

Change in appetite

Change in Sleep Pattern

It is common for depression and anxiety to be present at the same time. Most doctors and other clinicians see a lot of both. Like anxiety, you can have a little or you can have a lot. Full blown clinical depression is a serious illness requiring medical treatment. I want to add these considerations:

Depression can be insidious. People can slide into depression without really understanding what is happening to them. Are you aware that something is wrong? Any clinician knows the basic symptoms of depression.

There are also easy to use self-assessments available on the internet such as the Beck Depression Inventory (BDI). Be cautious though of self-diagnosis. People tend to score high when experiencing situational stress. What self-assessments may do for you is provide an objective indication that something is wrong.

Depression can be disguised by maladaptive behavior; forms of "self-medicating", including substance abuse, high risk activities or high risk sexual behaviors.

Depression is as physical as it is mental; many experience predominantly physical symptoms. These can feel like flu symptoms with temperature fluxes, aches and sweats. This is why having a medical provider on the support team is important.

Depression is often experienced and displayed differently by men and women, and among generations.

Like all mood disorders depression can show up when you least expect it; in other words, when "everything is going good".

Serious depression is correlated with suicide, *cardiovascular* illness and other forms of malaise. Like any other illness it can make you sick or kill you.

Depression is treatable. Yes, it takes work but we have the technology. There are many approaches involving medication, exercise and therapy that have been proven effective.

Therapy

Cognitive Behavioral Therapy (CBT)

> *People don't just get upset.*
> *They contribute to their upsetness.*
> *Albert Ellis*

CBT, an amalgam of Behavior Therapy and Cognitive Psychology, has been developed over the past thirty years into a well-researched, commonly used and accessible form of psychotherapy. I find it helpful for people who are seeking tools to help manage extreme emotions. I don't see CBT as better than any other form of therapy but its prevalence allows us to examine it as a good example of the therapeutic process.

My CBT joke...

A man is driving in a remote area at night. It is late, around 3 am. Suddenly he gets a flat tire. He stops, looks in his trunk and finds a spare tire but not a jack. Looking around him he notices a farmhouse on a hill. He thinks that the farmer might have a jack and starts up the hill intending to ask him. As he walks he is thinking: "The farmer is not going to like being woken up at 3 am. It's pretty embarrassing being in this situation. The farmer will probably think I am an idiot from the city and start chirping on me. That will be humiliating. Things will get worse. The farmer will get mad; he'll be yelling and screaming, the dog will be barking, I'll be humiliated and then he probably won't give me that jack".

The man knocks on the door.

The farmer opens the door and asks: "Can I help you?"

The man (angry) says: "I don't want your goddamn jack".

Most of my clients have been forced to hear that joke at one time. I like it because it so clearly illustrates the core principle of cognitive therapy. Life throws things at us every day; good, bad or horrible, but it is not the events themselves that create the emotions but the tendency of our thoughts to escalate from straightforward and reasonable to a place of distortion. Sure the farmer might not like getting up at 3 am (mind you, we don't know for sure he isn't already up) but will it really turn into a crazy conflict with a barking dog? That's possible but it is a distortion. Furthermore, is there some sort of rule that the driver has to feel humiliation in those circumstances? It wouldn't be a good thing if the farmer got mad but why would it follow that the driver needs to experience any particular emotional response?

RICHARD SCHWINDT

> *According to most studies, people's number one fear is public speaking. Number two is death. Death is number two! Does that sound right? This means to the average person, if you go to a funeral, you're better off in the casket than doing the eulogy.*
> *Jerry Seinfeld*

Carly

Carly likes to have a good time. She is the personification of fun in the sun. She's a travel agent who loves the free trips and is loved by her friends, co-workers and clients. Her carefree persona is quite fitting for her work. On her last trip to Jamaica she fainted while playing volleyball. She was okay after a bit but back in Canada she waited a few weeks then spoke to her family doctor. He was concerned and sent her for blood tests and an electrocardiogram. Shortly after she found herself having an angiogram, then seeing a cardiologist who recommended surgery for a weakening valve.

Carly's world turned upside down. She had no idea what was about to happen and began to obsess over everything. Would her decision to put off seeing a doctor kill her? Would the treatment hurt? How big would the scar be? Should she change her diet? And what about the drinking and partying? Stupid, stupid, stupid.

Now Carly can't sleep and can barely face work. She has lost ten pounds. She worries about all of this too because she needs – has to be – healthy. Her boyfriend tries to comfort her but his girlfriend is a good time girl; not this anxious drama queen. He cuts out leaving Carly with more to obsess over.

Thoughts stay with you. What did I do to deserve this? Why did my friends abandon me? You may even have extreme and disturbing thoughts of harming yourself. Every time these thoughts come back, whether you are aware of it or not, they affect your mood and body. Some of these thoughts are painful but true *("I should have seen a doctor sooner.")* and others are possible but unlikely. (*"What if no guy will want anything to do with me now?"*) Either way, they become increasingly distorted and consuming.

So pause here for a moment. How are Carly's thoughts making her feel? What triggers her? Maybe seeing an attractive healthy woman, hearing about heart disease on TV or looking at a poster of a southern island. She can learn to manage these thoughts and prevent much of the hurt and distress they cause. Heart disease changed her story and she can change it back. In fact she can make it better. It will require work but the process of changing your thoughts is well understood.

Many approaches to therapy address negative thinking. Most workbooks on depression and anxiety teach you skills, methods and formats for recording, assessing and changing your thoughts. This will help you investigate cognitive distortions and change them into thoughts that affirm and support you. Let's take the two examples:

"Did my decision to put off seeing a doctor kill me?"

This thought bears further examination. Likely it would have been good to see a doctor earlier but was the procrastination sufficient to kill her? Starting with the obvious, she is not dead yet. Neither does she yet have all the information provided during the diagnostic process. Heart disease can have serious consequences but it is also treatable. Carly's death is *possible* but so is the chance that through her actions (seeking diagnosis and treatment) she will survive. She is young and otherwise healthy. She has confidence in the medical provider. She can investigate the scenarios that lead to successful outcomes.

"No guy will want me after this."

No one would wish CHD on Carly but to this point she has lived a pretty charmed life. She is now thinking seriously about life, healing and people she has known with heart problems. The trigger is unfortunate but she is in a process of maturation. While most people think she's attractive she might take a deeper look at what makes her attractive as a human being. She might also ask herself about the kind of partner she wants in her life, surely not the guy who cuts and runs at the first sign of trouble. She may find that not only are guys still attracted to her but that she is in line for a more fulfilling relationship.

The deeper your commitment to the truth about yourself, the greater the gain. You will see the direct link between your thoughts, your emotions and physical well-being. The basic principle behind cognitive therapy is easy to understand; intervening between the situation at hand and your emotional response is a thought or thoughts.

Situation: The doctor tells Carly that they are going to do surgery.

Emotional response: Carly feels fear, sadness and isolation.

A CBT therapist would ask her to explore the thoughts that came to mind automatically. So the outcome might look like this:

Situation: The doctor tells Carly that they are going to do surgery.

Thought: "Then I will find out that it is worse than I thought. There will be an ugly scar. No one is going to want to be with me through this."

Emotion: Carly feels fear, sadness and isolation.

These thoughts are loaded emotionally. One in particular: *"Then I will find out that it is worse than I thought."*- is particularly charged, or the "hot" thought. This is probably what is known as a "cognitive distortion" - a thought that is distorted to the point where it no longer reflects an accurate view of reality. Most cognitive distortions represent possible scenarios but they do not represent necessary or even likely scenarios.

Your therapist may send you off to investigate the rational basis for your thoughts and evidence for and against them. In her office upon your return visit you will examine the evidence together.

Carly may discover that a weakening heart valve can usually be treated successfully. She may find someone else who has gone through the same experience. She might find out that her boyfriend did not represent all her social network; in fact, her friends, brother and parents are there to support her. It might look like this:

The rational thought: This situation is painful but recovery is a possibility if I commit to approaching this problem in a healthy way. And I am not alone; I have people who love me and are there for me. Also there are more community resources available than I thought; I guess lots of people have gone through this before.

Emotion: The negative emotions don't necessarily vanish but they may be reduced and displaced by a growing sense of optimism for your possibilities.

CBT therapists like to measure things. For example, she might have previously asked the client above to rate her fear out of 100. The client might be surprised that the fear might have started at 95% but by changing her thoughts the fear rating had gone down to 65%. This accomplishes two things; the fear is reduced and the client through her work and activity, has demonstrated that she has the *agency* to reduce that fear.

Changing your thinking does change your emotions and behaviors. Moreover, CBT can be applied to any situation in life where emotion get the better of you.

Ten best ridiculous Cognitive Distortions. Could these happen to you?

I am responsible for stuff I have nothing to do with. Today it's raining. It must be me!

This guy gave me a hard time is therefore a #@!& and I am therefore a saint (or is it the other way around?)

I should do this and I ought to think that; I really should!

I feel wrong therefore I must be wrong.

I made a mistake; I don't tolerate mistakes so I expect the world to collapse any minute.

I predict this is all going to end badly because I just know what she is thinking in that mean little brain of hers.

I get that my wife, kids, friends, extended family and the people I have worked with before really like me but my boss doesn't so I must be a terrible person.

This morning my husband said he loved me and then he hugged me, and the kids gave me a hug too and wished me a great day but I forgot to pass the peanut butter when Kyle asked; they really must hate me now!

Twenty people gave me a warm hello today but Bill ignored me - when did the world become such a rude place?

If I leave my job before I have a full pension it is only a matter of time until I am alone and cold, a pathetic ninety year old selling pencils on the street.

Good CBT therapists are fun and tend towards a robust sense of humor. They are present focused; not particularly interested in the past. They may exploit the absurdity of your cognitive distortions and automatic thoughts in the "C" part of CBT. In the "B" part they may have even more fun if they encourage you towards an experimental or investigative mind set.

They might use exposure therapy to help you find a way to face frightening situations or return to frightening contexts. They may also send you out to practice social skills on strangers or ask questions of distant family members. They put you out in front of the issues, treating problems as opportunities and your emotions as the subject at hand. They understand the plasticity of the brain and know yours can be retrained. They are like physical trainers who focus on the brain. I use stories, YouTube videos and other fun things to illustrate ideas.

Here is a story I use to illustrate CBT approaches and make a little fun of myself. Humour always anchors learning so I usually try to play it for a few laughs.

Bumping into you on the street as told to my client, Jon Green

Jon Green is my client and I tell him my CBT story.

Jon, this takes place three months in the future after you and I have completed counseling. It involves you, me and my therapist. On this day I am walking down the street, coming to the office to do a session. I am thinking about my session but feel a brush on the shoulder. I turn and see you walking away in the other direction. I continue here to do my session but I don't do a good session. Afterwards I ask myself what's wrong. Why was I so distracted?

I am self-aware of my thoughts and feelings

Then I remember running into you. So why does that bother me? I think about it and come up with two explanations: one, "That Jon sure is a rude guy!" and "I must be losing it as a therapist; I did such a lousy job that Jon doesn't even want to say hello on the street."

I articulate possible explanations for my thoughts and feelings.

This upsets me and I decide to speak to my therapist.

I consult with someone I trust.

49

I go to her office and tell her that I bumped into a client on the street and he didn't say hello, and that I thought he was either a rude guy or I was a terrible therapist. So she says to me: "Richard, are there any other possible explanations?"

So I say, "Well, I suppose it's possible he didn't see me, and it is also possible I looked busy and he didn't want to interrupt me."

We expand the possible explanations.

"Excellent Richard; now you have four possible explanations including two that are pretty innocent. So what is the evidence for each explanation?"

"Evidence, okay, Jon is a rude person; well he was never rude when I saw him as a client so I have no evidence. I am a terrible therapist; no therapist is perfect but over the years the feedback has been good so there's not much evidence for that. He didn't see me; well if I hadn't turned when I did I wouldn't have seen him - so there is some evidence for that. And as for not interrupting; I know I did look preoccupied so yes there is evidence for that too."

We examine the evidence for each explanation

"So the evidence tends to support the more innocent explanation."

We move our support towards the explanation with the best evidence.

"Yes, but it is still bothering me."

We adopt an investigative mind set.

"Do you ever do follow up phone calls?"

"Yes."

"Why don't you phone him up and investigate what really happened today."

So I go to the phone and call you up and likely discover that you either didn't see me or you didn't want to interrupt me...

We have now addressed my worries effectively and decisively.

But there is another possibility...

I pick up the phone, call you and you say: "Yes, I did see you Richard but you were a lousy therapist, didn't help me at all and I don't want to waste another minute on you," (sound of phone hanging up).

Now I am devastated. I rush back to my therapist and say: "The worst was true! He was rude on the phone and I am a lousy therapist!"

Sometimes the most feared explanation is true. We can still use the process to address new information.

"Richard, how many follow ups did you do this week?"

"Maybe ten."

"And they all told you that you did a bad job?"

"No, just this guy."

"How many have you done over the years?"

"Hundreds, thousands."

"And every week someone tells you that you are a bad therapist?"

"No."

"So why then are you elevating this guy to a point where you label yourself a lousy therapist, other than the fact that it happened today? Maybe he had a bad day or maybe you didn't help him. If you are feeling brave you could always call him back and find out, but it is a cognitive distortion to give this individual the responsibility for your esteem as a therapist."

> *Therapy is not really an act of love, and there is a danger in being too friendly and loving. At times therapy comes closer to being an act of aggression, in which the therapist joins forces with whatever sanity there is in the patient or the family and then beats up on the pathology. I love my patient, in the same way that Michelangelo loved marble—if I keep chipping away I can free what I see inside.*
> *Frank Pittman*

What do you find a little scary to contemplate? And what do you find terrifying? In the Cognitive Behavioral Therapy world people make lists and then quantify them.

Meet Jamie

Six month ago Jamie and Ellen were at a party. As with their usual arrangement, it was Jamie's turn to have a few drinks and Ellen's turn to drink Perrier and lime then drive home. They had a good time and while on route home Ellen suddenly became unable to breathe, panicked, fainted and drove off the road, wrecking the car and giving herself a concussion.

The time since has been a nightmare. Ellen is unable to work; she has been to what seems like endless rounds of medical visits and she has experienced severe headaches, dizziness, nausea and erratic moods. Ellen was diagnosed with a faulty valve and told that she will need to go on medication and likely prepare for heart surgery. Their children, aged 14 and 15, were terrified by the news and the changes in their parents. Jamie has been tearful and consumed with guilt. He keeps telling Ellen that he should have been driving that night, which only makes her angry because their arrangement had worked fine for years and his contention somehow suggests she was at fault for not knowing she was going to faint.

That's not how Jamie meant it. He would have preferred to be injured himself before seeing his wife suffer like this. And worse, in a household with two busy teenagers neither of them can drive. There is a medical restriction on Ellen and since the accident Jamie is too anxious. Every time he tried to drive he has literally felt his body begin to freeze up, experiencing a deep numbing and dissociation.

Jamie has been working with a CBT therapist to overcome his anxiety. They have used a number of tactics to determine the best approach. In particular, they have looked at some of the irrational thoughts and beliefs effecting Jamie. For example:

Ellen had always been healthy; there was no indication prior that she was having any problems. Jamie has the irrational idea that he should have somehow known what was coming.

Jamie and Ellen had a responsible designated driver plan in place for years. There is no reason to believe that if he had been driving home and she had suddenly had trouble breathing the crash would not have happened.

The unpredictability of certain events exacerbates the chances of increased anxiety. Someone could drive for a lifetime without fainting and then it could just happen. Jamie's therapist asked him to write a list of things that he fears. This is Jamie's list:

Driving

Driving on the highway

Showing signs of anxiety or nervousness publicly

Showing nervousness at work

Losing his job

Losing confidence in all aspects of life

Crying in public

Excessive sweating

Peeing himself

Getting sick or sicker

Not being able to go out in public

People laughing at him

People thinking he is weak

Being asked: "Why aren't you driving?" by a casual acquaintance

Having to go back to the site of the accident for some reason

Having the police decide that the accident is somehow his fault and arresting him

Hearing that a rumour is being spread about you in town

Ellen becoming disabled

Ellen suddenly dying

Not being able to go to appointments with Ellen

The kids falling apart

The kids using drugs/having inappropriate sex/failing at school

Not experiencing pleasure

Never having sex with Ellen again

Sudden increase in past phobia (heights, spiders, etc.)

Not being able to be alone

Dying suddenly of a heart attack or stroke

*When we write a list we objectify our thoughts and take some agency over them. The next step was to rank his thoughts. He decided that in his scale **one** was "I'm not too worried." and **ten** was "Worst scenario!"*

One

Sudden increase in past phobia (heights, spiders, etc.)

Not being able to be alone

Having the police decide that the accident is somehow his fault and arresting him

Two

Never having sex with Ellen again

Not experiencing pleasure

Three

Dying suddenly of a heart attack or stroke

Four

Not being able to go to appointments with Ellen

Five

Hearing that a rumour is being spread about you in town

Six

Driving

Driving on the highway

Showing signs of anxiety or nervousness publicly

Showing nervousness at work

Seven

The kids falling apart

The kids using drugs/having inappropriate sex/ failing at school

Eight

Ellen becoming disabled

Not being able to go out in public

People laughing at him

People thinking he is weak

Nine

Being asked: "Why aren't you driving?" by a casual acquaintance

Having to go back to the site of the accident for some reason

Ten

Ellen leaving him

Ellen suddenly dying

Jamie feels shamed by his choices. The part of him that believes that he should be strong is embarrassed that the fear of losing his wife comes ahead of concerns about the kids. He believes it is egocentric to put himself first. Similarly, his fear of embarrassment is itself embarrassing to him; making him feel again like he is more concerned with his ego than the people he loves.

These choices can be explored and Jamie can be led towards forgiving himself for thinking of himself. I sometimes remind clients that there is such a thing as the *'realpolitik of the mind'*.

If you are travelling with children and air pressure falls on a plane they tell you to put your own oxygen mask on first. We can frame Jamie's self-care as a pragmatic choice necessary for the highest functioning member of the family.

He might look at the evidence for and against the idea that Ellen would either die or leave him. Were there other possibilities? Maybe she will remain well with treatment. What exactly are the chances that she will die? Has she even had any thoughts through this crisis of leaving the man who is holding her up?

His therapist might ask him to explore the idea that he is somehow required to be ashamed if he thinks about his own needs. We want to do our best when loved ones struggle but is there a rule book somewhere that says we have to be saints at the same time?

We want Jamie to be the detective; not sitting around waiting for disaster but actively exploring the alleged disaster and acting on it. He might find my ideas funny or think I am a crazy therapist but in the end it is likely that the fear of Ellen dying/leaving has somehow found itself demoted from ten to four. That may give him some agency with other items on the list, now that he has dealt with the toughest.

People have a terrible time with their worst fear. They avoid and avoid because they are overwhelmed. Taking on and addressing that fear leaves them with a powerful sense of having accomplished something difficult.

Exposure approaches

> *Men go to far greater lengths to avoid what*
> *they fear than to obtain what they desire.*
> *Dan Brown*

Expose yourself to your deepest fear; after that,
fear has no power, and the fear of freedom
shrinks and vanishes. You are free.
Jim Morrison

Exposure therapy can be incredibly effective and quick. It comes in three basic forms:

Graduated exposure: In this approach the therapist and client work together to gradually begin exposure to the things or activities that frighten them.

Flooding: Intensive full exposure to the source of the fear. American Psychiatrist David Burns writes about asking people phobic of elevators to get in the elevator outside his office and come out when they are cured.

Imaginal exposure: In this approach the source of the fear is approached in someone's imagination or through hypnosis. This would be commonly be used where real exposure is not possible (e.g. a sexual assault).

Let's go back to Jamie who is too anxious to drive. If it was me using graduated exposure to treat him I might start by having him state his intention to drive again. Then I might ask him to imagine a time in the past where he enjoyed driving or being in a car. Perhaps a fun trip with laughter and an exciting destination. I want to re-associate a strong pleasant emotion with driving.

We might have him start by sitting in the car in the driveway. He might feel silly about this. In fact feeling silly might trip the absurdity of the situation in his mind. I might even suggest he sit there saying "zoom zoom".

This might progress to having him drive up and down in the driveway with his kids saying: "zoom zoom". The more laughing or even cursing the therapist the better.

So you are thinking: *This is a tragedy; there has been hurt and injury, why are you treating it like a joke?* Recall that Mr. Anxiety wants you to take him seriously. And as long as Jamie thinks of his car as a rolling death trap he is going to remain anxious.

Jamie is strongly motivated to drive the car and some interesting things might happen here including him saying: *"I need to drive; not have some therapist make a monkey out of me. I'm going to pick up some milk."* Like most therapists, I am a little arrogant and don't really care what you think of me, provided you get better.

Another possible scenario is that Jamie decides this is ridiculous and quits therapy, waits a few weeks then says to himself: *"I don't need some therapist to teach me how to drive, I'm just going to do it."* When Jamie signalled his intent to get better it set in motion many psychological and spiritual mechanisms of healing.

Or we may just finish the process so that Jamie is able to drive down the street again.

Be creative and remember to flow *into your fear...*

Hidden emotions

Samantha's father was a high achieving perfectionist. As she grew up Samantha was constantly challenged to "do better" but it seemed like nothing she ever achieved met her father's expectations. He seemed oblivious to the fact that having CHD made everything more difficult for her. As she went through life she found herself constantly trying to meet the expectations of others. Her husband found this frustrating.

He wished she would lighten up on herself and relax with him. He was frankly sick of his "perfect" wife. She was always nice but fretted about him, the kids and work.

One day while Samantha was out walking she had a dizzy spell. It was so intense that she had to be assisted home by a passerby. At the hospital they performed an electrocardiogram and an echocardiogram. The cardiology resident told her that nothing had changed and her condition seemed stable. Had she been under more stress lately? Samantha seemed to shrug it off but withdrew further into herself and set to work cleaning, working overtime and worrying about everyone but herself.

One night her husband confronted her. He didn't want a withdrawn cleaning machine; he wanted a wife and a partner. If she didn't deal with his behavior he was going to leave. He wanted a reaction from her – any reaction – but she just went into the bedroom and closed the door.

I often see the Samantha's of the world in my office. They are nice hard working people and don't quite understand why they do the things they do or why people respond to them with frustration. They get a little frustrated sometimes but put it back inside and carry on. Samantha's father is not a bad guy; *his* father grew up poor during the depression when hard work and a stiff upper lip were necessary for survival. And if you have CHD then all the more reason to work hard and put your emotions to the side.

David Burns and Gabor Mate are both physicians who have written on the psychological and physical consequences of chronically repressing an accurate emotional response to the people and world around you. They both purport that we experience emotion for a reason and if we suppress our responses we put ourselves at risk. This might be the caregiver who always puts herself second to others or the person who meets life's stressors with denial.

I sometimes tell my clients about the 100 pound brick. Drop it on your foot and you'll probably yell, swear or jump up and down from pain. You don't say, "Oh don't worry I'm never bothered by a large brick on my foot". And yet with the psychological 100 pound brick people often deny that the event behind it has any effect. To me, psychological events conform to the laws of physics every bit as much as material events.

Psychotherapy can be particularly helpful for this kind of anxiety. If Samantha was in my office I might try to guide her towards engaging in her real feelings which could include anger at her father, terror that her heart is deteriorating or understanding her husband's desire to have her in his emotional life.

The point wouldn't be to lock her in anger so much as connect her to the constellation of emotions shared by human beings and allow herself to feel.

I am only scratching the surface of CBT. There are some excellent books listed in the resources list at the end of the book.

Narrative

Think about the stories that define your life. Here is one I tell in my office:

Ruth had a pacemaker implant and was told to take it easy for a week by the surgeon. This was during a snowy week in the winter and she was grateful to stay home with a book. A few days after the surgery her daughter Felicia asked if she could take the car to visit a friend for coffee. Ruth agreed but warned her to drive carefully. About twenty minutes after she left the phone rang and Felicia reported that she had been in an accident and needed her mother there. Ruth dressed, got into the other car and went to the accident site, where she saw an ambulance, police car and fire truck. She couldn't park close by so she had to wade through snow to the site and arrived sweaty and breathless. She discovered that Felicia had slid across traffic into a car in the other lane. No one was hurt. The other car had been banged into the ditch. The entire front end of Ruth's Mazda was caved in. Two stories came into her mind:

Story one: Ruth was close to her mother, and when she died a few years back Ruth had been devastated. Her mother wasn't affluent but had a new Mazda which she left to her only daughter. Now, in a moment of reckless stupidity Felicia had wrecked that car, endangered herself and the other driver. Not to mention putting her mother's recovery at risk.

Story two: Cars are machines used for transportation. Everyone is safe, the car is insured and on a slippery road this could have happened to anyone. There are reasons to be grateful. She can go to bed when she gets home and continue her recovery and rest.

It is important to note that both of these versions are true. But story one will leave Ruth sad about her mother and angry at Felicia. This will make for conflict between them and leave Ruth with a strong sense of loss.

A car accident isn't a good thing but story two recognizes the reality that life can throw difficult and unexpected events at us. We need to build our responses into an accurate narrative, but one that allows us to function and act on tasks ahead of us.

Don Miguel Ruiz, in his wonderful book *The Four Agreements*, says that our words - written, spoken or thought – are white or black magic. They are powerful influences on our vision and response to the world.

What kind of story do you tell about yourself and your heart?

"…mine is a tragic tale of…"

or

"…life is full of struggles but there remain so many reasons for gratitude…"

Psychiatric Medication

If you have CHD or are emotionally effected by someone who does, the question of medication may arise for management of stress, anxiety or depression. You may be thinking *"Great, that's what I need – more drugs."* There are other alternatives for emotional management. That said, they are an option that may need to be explored.

Most therapists note the effectiveness of therapy while pointing out the absence of unpleasant side effects and the acquisition of skills that can be used over a lifetime. But sometimes taking medication is helpful. I am not a doctor and do not recommend medication to people. However, for some of my clients I note there are medications available and recommend they discuss them with a physician.

Their responses vary from: *"Wow, there are drugs for this!"* to *"I would never violate this temple with chemicals from the pharma-industrial complex."* Some have taken meds before and others have never considered them. I am a pragmatist and favour the shortest line between the problem and recovery. Some people with severe emotional struggles can swallow a pill when they can't do much else.

The meds are not going to change the upcoming surgery but they may help you cope. Do your homework and talk to your doctor. Remember that medications have a generic or scientific name, as well as a brand name. While the scientific name is consistent the brand name may vary in different jurisdictions. For example, the Selective Serotonin Reuptake Inhibitor (SSRI) Escitalopram is also called Cipralex in Canada and Lexapro in the United States.

Anti-depressants are not addictive but they have some side effects and many have withdrawal issues. They are obviously used for depression but are often the drug of choice for anxiety as well. Both depression and anxiety are mood disorders - they are different - but the medication seems to work for both. There are different classes and generations of anti-depressants.

Benzodiazepines (e.g. Lorazepam/Ativan) provide short term relief from anxiety or stress, and are often used as a sleep aid but they are risky for long term use, a bad combo with alcohol and can be addictive. They are sometimes offered prior to cardiac procedures to help you through the fear.

People sometimes wonder if they are going to turn into zombies or experience a personality change. For the vast majority of people properly prescribed, (and taken as prescribed), medication will address the symptoms directly. I take Cipralex from time to time and I remain "me", just without the anxiety symptoms.

Psychiatric meds behave differently with different people. Cipralex works well for me but might leave someone else with side effects or little symptom relief. You should discuss with your doctor whether any particular medication is working for you or not. It is also important to understand most anti-depressants take six to eight weeks to reach full effect. In addition many of the side effects are short term and will disappear over a few weeks. Your doctor may ask you to hang in for a bit to see if they subside.

The most common ongoing side effects with current anti-depressants are sexual side effects. Before you panic remember not everyone is affected the same way or at all. Some of my clients have been on an SSRI's for years and are surprised when I mention the sex thing. If this becomes a problem speak to your doctor; there are some compensatory meds and some anti-depressants that have little or no effect on sexual function.

Remember your special circumstances. Medications can interact with each other. Exercise agency and make sure that your doctor and pharmacist are aware of the implications of the mix. Some antidepressants can effect cardiac rhythm.

Children and teens

Fear isn't so difficult to understand. After all, weren't we all frightened as children? Nothing has changed since Little Red Riding Hood faced the big bad wolf. What frightens us today is exactly the same sort of thing that frightened us yesterday. It's just a different wolf. This fright complex is rooted in every individual.
Alfred Hitchcock

When trailers for the movie *2012* appeared, I was approached by a colleague regarding kids who had become frightened that the world was really going to end in 2012.

Commercials for industrial safety have upset numerous kids ("Don't be the next worker cut in half on the job!"). Some kids have anxious parents who for various reasons worry, try to control, and fear the world. Kids are also expected to perform at home, in the school yard, competitive sports, etc. And of course kids worry about their parents.

No one should be surprised that there are more anxious kids in general. The world is not less safe than it used to be; quite the contrary. And the focus on kid's safety, while overdone at times has doubtless saved many from abuse, injury and death. But my generation of parents and those since, have often hovered over kids trying to protect them from harm, real and imagined.

All kids are different. I was a laid back bookish kid with a quirky sense of humour. My grandson, Griffin on the other hand, just won the energy award in preschool. When my grandkids are on their way over, I usually tell my wife that *"Hurricane Griffin is blowing into town."*

This raises an interesting point to anyone who spends time with children. Yes, we can assess their family history and functioning and we can assess and measure things like language, processing, intelligence, developmental milestones but all children are individuals. They have their own temperaments. Sure they can be affected by CHD, but each one has unique affinities; sometimes of mysterious origin.

Alex and Emma loved canoeing on the lake, watercolours and supporting the eco-system. Their son, almost from the start, was fascinated by competitive body contact sports, the more intense the better.

I told Alex and Emma to relax with the son who seemed to have been born into the wrong family. Lots of people in this world have that particular affinity and someday they might be grateful when they need someone to do the heavy lifting.

Children take their messaging from you. They will look to you and respond to your mood and tone, no matter the overt message you are trying to portray. If there is one idea I try to impress upon parents in counselling it is that, whatever they say or do, the children are taking cues from you.

How do the other children in the family get the attention and support they need? What if they have their own challenges?

Erin was so preoccupied with her younger son's illness that when her older son was sent home from school she became furious. She flew into a rage and told him: "I have enough going on with your brother – I don't have time for this."

I learn much from counselling kids. I enjoy it because one significant strength most kids have is a sense of fun and wonder. A kid having fun is a child who is learning. That makes sessions fun by necessity. I typically see kids with their parents and bring them in on the fun. The need for a child to be a child is critical.

Kids need play, school, friends, regular expectations, responsibilities, meals and bedtime. They also need appropriate boundaries and discipline, engaged parents and restrictions on access to media. Teenagers need all of the above with a gradual relaxation of boundaries and increase in privileges.

There are extremes of strictness and permissiveness and lots of room in between. Two parents often are not on the same page. This is not damaging to a child provided parents caucus, share and sort out differences. Kids are quite resilient.

Some kids are born with some anxiety in their temperament but many face situations that create anxiety as well. To a certain extent they will have their response influenced by their parents but some things are plain scary; such as:

Trying to function with an undiagnosed or unaddressed learning disability

Schoolyard bullying

Rejection by friends

Parental separation

Physical, psychological, sexual abuse

Witnessing abuse

Parental substance abuse

An invasive medical test

Death or illness of a parent or sibling

Television report of terrorism or environmental catastrophe

Animal bite

Bee or wasp sting

Getting lost

Struggling in the water

Falling out of a tree

For teenagers you might add:

A painful fight with a friend

A bad breakup

Bad first sexual experience

Bad first driving experience

Bad first experience with alcohol or drugs

Cyberbullying

Notable physical differences from peers (taller, shorter, skinnier, fatter, early or late sexual maturation) or perception that they are different from others.

A few of these things are part of the normal passage into adulthood and may seem easy to dismiss. However, they will be experienced differently by different children. Something that seems minor to a parent may be a very big deal to a child or teen. You may be indifferent during the latest TV report on the Ozone layer while your child watches in horror.

So now we come to the child with CHD, not forgetting the sibling of a child with CHD or the child who has a parent with CHD.

Brent started to work at a burger place when he was 16. He went to work on the day of his father's heart surgery. His boss sent him home for the day after he found him crying in the lunchroom.

Learning to manage fear, conflict and adversity is a normal part of childhood. Maturation involves gradually encountering the challenges of the world and developing the ability to function in it. Parents, teachers and peers play a significant role in guiding this process.

Kids with CHD may lose time to tests, procedures, surgery and recovery. They may not be able to play team sports or bond with other kids in the same way as others.

Anxious kids may show it in different ways, bearing in mind that the tendency to withdraw from anxiety is the same, whether it occurs in an adult or a child. A child may withdraw from friends, school, mealtimes, family activities, vacations, outings; all the things kids would normally be doing.

Angry kids might lash out at others or behave irrationally or in a way that undermines themselves.

Just as with adults strong emotions may be masked. Younger kids might use tantrums, crying, complaining of a tummy ache, picking on a sibling to show their fear. Teens may engage in cutting their skin, pulling out their own hair, isolating themselves, refusing food, substance abuse or dressing strangely. Seriously traumatized kids may dissociate and withdraw into themselves.

Children need agency and communion as much as their parents. Supporting their ability to influence events and come up with strategies is powerful. As well, their continuing engagement with family, extended family and other children keeps them *flowing into their anxiety.*

Some examples:

Ten year old Sherry refused to go to school. Her parents were baffled; she always liked school. They asked her if something had happened. She went into her room and refused to come out. She also refused to eat, she said her stomach hurt. Sherry's mother called the principal to ask if something had happened. The principle had no idea but said she would check with the teacher and some of the children. Upon investigation, one of Sherry's classmates said that they had told Sherry that she was too weak and puffing all the time and therefore was no longer allowed to play with the other girls.

Fourteen year old Dylan was confident and happy. One day, for no reason he could discern, two older boys surrounded him, pushed him to the ground and started kicking him. He tried to run away but the other boys caught him easily. He suffered bruising and two broken ribs. His parents were horrified and the police were called. Both boys were caught and charged but Dylan changed. He lost his effervescence, quit going to the after school club and adopted new friends who introduced him to marijuana.

Naomi, 8, and her sister Jenna, 9, were taken to a restaurant by their parents for dinner. They were excited and happy until their parents told them that even though they still loved them they no longer loved each other. They would always be there for them but they were going to live in different homes. Jenna seemed totally unaffected by the news, as if she hadn't heard it at all. Naomi was mortified and was by turns angry, whiny, sad and behaviorally immature towards her mother who she blamed. Shortly after Jenna's CHD symptoms increased dramatically.

As parents we have this idea that we can protect our kids and, given the right home environment, raise healthy well-adjusted young people. This is true, but only up to a point. Bad things can happen to any child, and any child for a variety of reasons can become anxious. Troubled kids can come from good homes. Frightening events may occur that parents never hear about.

CHD in the family doesn't mean that any of these things are going happen or that you are going to have a troubled child. But it is not a *good* thing and it does force everyone to adapt. The adaptations can be helpful and wise, or dysfunctional.

Jeffrey learned early how to communicate well and help others feel good about themselves. He made lots of friends and even though he couldn't keep up to others in sports and games he was always included.

Nina tried to keep up with the other children playing soccer at school. After a day when she threw up on the field Nina felt different from the other children and humiliated. She decided that going out, taking risks and getting close to people was dangerous.

Adaptations made in childhood can last a lifetime. It is not too far a stretch to think that Jeffrey might find adult life easier than Nina.

That said, kids from good homes have protective factors and advantages. Let's go back and look at how Jenna's parents responded to her emotions. Clearly their separation is going to effect the kids. Their daughters have felt the tension for months without understanding what was going on. As it turns out Jenna's mom met another man and will be eventually be moving in with him. Jenna's mom is consumed with guilt, particularly as she witnesses Jenna struggle. Jenna's Dad is torn between anger and sadness. Sometimes he can't help but think: *she is going to make Jenna sicker than she is.* This is not a good time for anyone in the family.

Both parents agreed they would do whatever they could for Jenna. As it turns out, Jenna's mom is seeing a counsellor and her Dad is seeing the pastor. They have started in the right place to address their own issues.

They have also resolved to put the kids first. This is not easy at all for them but it means they can share notes without Dad saying "you created this problem", and mom saying "If you had been a good husband." They start by continuing to assure both girls that their lives will mostly go on as usual; they will see their pets, go to their school and keep their friends. They back this up by arranging for the girls to have some fun, see friends and helping them with homework. They continue to have expectations for chores, bedtimes, homework, etc.

They go for family therapy at a local family services agency. The therapist allows everyone to talk and share their emotions. The girls learn that they can do this safely with their parents and that Naomi is able to admit that she is mad at her mom. This emotion is validated and allowed on the basis that her mother shares responsibility for care and discipline with Dad. Dad backs up mom.

The girls don't yet know about the other man but are practising good communication with their mom. She is able to tell them that she has met another man and that in time she will introduce him.

Those who have spent time with separating couples know that this is a best case scenario. It rarely goes this smoothly. What is key here is that both parents are trying to use the support available and consider what is happening from their kid's point of view. You can use most counselling techniques with kids but there are a few rules that help the process.

Communicating with young people means adjusting your messaging to their developmental stage. There are concepts that very young children don't understand. Similarly, older teens do not like being talked down to.

Mike went into Dean's room and counted his pills. He discovered that Dean had missed a few doses. He angrily confronted his 15 year old son when he arrived home.

"Why are you being so stupid? If you miss your meds you will get sick again and land back in hospital!"

"Dad, stop talking to me like I am 8. I'm 15 and I can handle this. I can take care of my own meds now."

Dean may in fact have missed his meds a few times and this does put him at risk of getting sick; his father's worst fear. Still Mike's tone was part of the problem. Psychiatrist Eric Berne created a schema for communication that suggested that our statements fit one of four tones:

Child statements

Oh, look at the puppy!

I am so happy for you!

Oh, come on, you promised.

Adult statements

Let's examine this situation together.

I want to go out at five.

There are several choices here.

Parent statements

I want you to check out this website.

You need to take a look at all your options.

You will feel better if you stop eating at night.

Critical Parent statements

You are being foolish and deserve to fail.

Stop saying those ridiculous things right now.

You would have passed the test if you hadn't wasted the night away.

Of course there are "tones" attached to these statements. And it is important to understand that none of these tones are wrong in of themselves. That said, it is the critical parent tone that typically creates the most problems. Dean feels stupid when his dad speaks as the critical parent and becomes defensive. He also is scared by the fearful undertone behind his father's angry response.

Mike feels frustrated because he is not reaching his son. He is also associating into unsettling memories of seeing his son in hospital and feeling that fear again. He might have had more success as a straightforward parent.

"Hey bud, I think you need to take these on a regular basis. I'd like you to start using one of those plastic containers with the days marked."

Or perhaps come across as helpful adult:

It must be hard to take these things every day. Do you think if we sit down together we can come up with a plan to help you remember?

It would be unwise for Mike to allow an 8 year old to handle his own meds. With a teenager prone to distraction it is a worry, but it is reasonable to expect that he can learn to manage them himself with support.

Alternately Mike could adopt a solution focused approach to helping Dean. Put simply, being human we tend to focus on the negative. Solution focused therapists do the opposite. They take success and especially agency and put their focus there. It allows kids to identify their successes and learn from them.

Mike: When is the last time you took your meds every day?

Dean: Last month when I went to Aunt Sue's I took them every day and was only late once.

Mike: Excellent! How did you do that?

Dean: I don't know. I just did.

Mike: I don't believe that. You did something smart and I am curious to know what it is.

Dean: The night table in the bedroom was right beside the bed so I put the pills there so I could see them.

Mike: Does it make a difference when you can actually see the pills?

Dean: I guess. It's funny, I remember the colours when I see them. The blue one and the green one.

Mike: I wonder if we could set up some sort of visual reminder for you.

Mike and Dean have figured out that Dean is visual in orientation and found a way to help him take his pills that fits for him. But Mike was able to suss this out by zeroing in on a success/solution and exploring from there. Dean did not feel that his dad was challenging or doubting him. On the contrary Dean felt like his dad was looking for the best in him.

Time is different for kids than it is for adults. You need to act quickly to help them. To give one example, in Ontario there are long wait times for psychological assessments in schools and children's mental health agencies, which in some cases might shed light on how anxiety effects learning or the existence of a learning/processing challenge. But there are also private psychologists who can do these assessments faster for a fee. Some parents have the means to pay a psychologist or budget it as a priority.

The developmental stages of childhood pass quickly and with the added burden of CHD children need to be encouraged in keeping on track.

Context and environment is the ultimate source of safety for kids, with a sidebar for culture and spirit. Home, family, friends, meals, bedtimes, school, expectations, chores compose a child's safe world.

Parents and family are by far the best supports for children and teens. I see kids for parts of sessions and I do sessions with teens; whenever possible I keep parents closely engaged in the process or do family therapy. The parents may not be cardiologists or child therapists but are the expert on their child.

Very young children are helped almost entirely through a combination of play and simple talk.

Teens can do well in counselling but they typically don't love sitting in a room talking about their feelings to a therapist they perceive as being much older. It helps if a particular therapist has an affinity for working with teens.

Helping kids develop skills in self-soothing and emotional management confers a lifetime advantage. If I see a young person who has learned CBT skills it is much easier for them to pick up and apply them to any stressful situation.

There are many ways to do this, including family discussions on life and the news that point out the importance of managing emotions well and intermittent but strong praise for moments when your child exhibits emotional maturity.

Justin was needlessly singled out by his teacher for making a mistake. He felt embarrassed but did not react or respond. Later, discussing this with his mother she noted that by controlling his emotions, putting the situation in perspective and processing it with her, he had demonstrated some wisdom and not allowed the situation to get worse.

Parents need to be empowered. Services for children and teens tend to be more political and bureaucratized than services for adults. They sometimes forget that children are thinking, feeling people and become preoccupied with diagnosis and assessment. Go after what your child needs. Get the best assessment and help you can access/afford.

Parents can become preoccupied with diagnosis and assessment too. And of course there are mentally ill and very troubled children and teens. That doesn't change the fact that they are struggling. You will always have to relate to them as people.

Children and teens can become suicidal. Like adults they can have passing thoughts, plan to harm themselves or execute attempts. The best defense is to stay engaged with them. Notice what they are writing, what they are watching on TV and what they are doing on the computer. If the topic comes up for any reason (something on TV or with a friend), keep it light but talk about it. Don't be afraid to ask, "Have you ever had thoughts of hurting yourself?" If you have worries don't hesitate to consult a professional or a crisis line. If your worries have some backing (e.g. a note or poem about death or suicide), don't let it slide; increase supervision, address it directly and get help right away. Better to feel dumb for overreacting than horrible for not acting on a real concern.

Cutting behaviours are not usually suicidal behaviours but they still emerge from emotional distress. Get your child help if they cut. It is a potentially addictive and disfiguring activity and it needs to be addressed directly.

Doctors, with good reason, are reluctant to medicate troubled kids. Do your homework and be a good consumer. Sometimes medication is needed to help a child manage, but be sure within yourself that the reason is sound. You might also want to consult a paediatrician or a child psychiatrist if medication is being considered.

Lighten up; Mr. Anxiety wants you to be sombre; a kid who is laughing and having fun is a less anxious kid.

Body image

Scars are tattoos with better stories.
From a Toyota advertisement in Sports Illustrated magazine

I thought I was the ugliest guy around when I was young and was astonished when a good looking Italian woman agreed to marry me. Years later I asked what had attracted her to me and she said, *"I thought you were handsome."* I still don't believe her. It is difficult for me to think of myself as anything but unattractive. However, the reality is that while I'll never give George Clooney a run for the money, I do fall within normal parameters for masculine appearance.

Our perception can be suggested to us. I read a medical report on me once that noted a "deformed left chest". I ran to a mirror and there it was. It was obvious but I had never noticed until I looked for it. Now I see it every time I look in the mirror.

My body is crossed with scars, especially the chest. That's why I admire a handsome masculine chest on the beach. It is not something that keeps me up at night but there have been times when it has bothered me; especially when I was younger.

Most serious heart defects are surgically repaired. And though the surgery has become less invasive over time, much of it still requires cutting through the sternum which is a particularly hard part of your skeleton. This can make for an impressive scar.

This can be particularly challenging to young women who may feel self-conscious about the scars, wondering if it affects how others see them, and a young woman with a scar may make clothing or brassiere choices to cover the scar. This does not mean they are less attractive but it does mean that both women and men with CHD may be acutely conscious that their body came with a factory defect.

The things that make you really attractive - healthy living, exercise, good food, joy, confidence are the real issue here. We may be unconsciously aware that reproductive choice is based on health. You may compare yourself with the best looking person you know or someone on television.

If we neglect ourselves, withdraw from life or ruminate over our cardiac issues, we will look less attractive.

Katrina met her first serious boyfriend in college. On the morning after their first night together, they went to breakfast. She quietly asked him if her scar bothered him. He looked confused for a moment then said, "There's a scar? I didn't see it."

Maybe there are people out there who will make an issue of a scar, but it is part of you. Do you really want to be with that person?

Remember that in cognitive behavioral therapy, we challenge our thoughts. We ask ourselves if our interpretation is accurate and whether that interpretation is affecting our thoughts and emotions.

Marital issues

> *He also kept schtum about heart surgery*
> *he had while Maria was pregnant.*
> *Arnold explained: 'That's the way I handle things. And*
> *it always has worked. But it's not the best thing for people*
> *around me because some information I just keep to myself.'*
> *Arnold Schwarzenegger quoted in Mail Online regarding*
> *surgery to repair faulty valve*

You have a spouse with CHD

Well, this can be scary. You love your partner but there are times where that love is put to the test. What can they do? What is going to make them sick or exhausted? What if you go on vacation and they get sick?

Your spouse with CHD is going to have times where they are not doing so well. And these times may not be predictable. It can be frustrating if they can't pull their weight at home or contribute to household income. There will be periods of recovery after surgery and medical procedures. Being ill can be a self-centred experience where your spouse may withdraw or become needy. This can take some of the fun out of life and add to your burden.

People who don't manage their emotions may internalize (withdrawal, depression, addiction), or they may externalize (anger, blame, controlling behaviors). If they are unable to self soothe, they may want you to be a receptacle for their emotions.

Carl was stomping around the house prior to getting a pacemaker. He yelled at the kids, and was up half the night. Helga finally had to tell him to settle down and remember that he lived with his family and needed to consider their feeling too.

Debbie was so depressed about the change in her heart status that she took to her bed and withdrew from family life. Glen finally had to tell her that though the news was upsetting but she was still needed.

It is for this reason that a direct line needs to be drawn between a person's experience of CHD and their emotional experience. We are, in the end, all responsible for managing our own emotions. This goes for you too. It is no fun waiting for hours in a hospital or by a bed. You may be terrified and confused by what is happening. You may not want to share those feelings with your spouse; instead putting up a front of cheerful optimism. This is where your social supports and maybe a therapist can help.

If you find yourself in the role of caregiver remember that the principle requirement for survival is balance. If you do not have respite, recreation and others to share the load, you will quickly become burned out and love will turn into resentment. Caregivers can also become sick themselves if they do not look after their own needs.

Know what is happening to your spouse. Know what medications he or she takes and remember that in an emergency you might be required to answer some questions about medical history. You will be much more helpful if you know the case history as well as she does. Take a CPR course together and know what you would do in an emergency.

It is not a fun conversation but you should have an idea what your spouse wants if there is a major deterioration in health and an end of life decision has to be made. All married couples need to address this eventually; you may need to address it sooner. And yes, having your will and power of attorney up to date is a good idea.

You have CHD and a spouse

Having a loving partner is a good thing and you need to keep him or her at the top of your mind. He is worried but he also has expectations. He will do his best but needs you to get better. There will be times where you need to do things when you still feel shaky, out of breath or tired. You have responsibilities and that is good. They motivate you and help keep you alive.

Talk to your spouse about your experience. Share important information about your health. This is not just your problem. It is his or hers as well. You may be the one having that procedure tomorrow but they have to be there too, waiting and scared. She may also have to take care of the kids and manage the household while you are out of commission.

A word about sex

If you are a regular movie watcher you may have seen a movie where someone with a heart problem succumbs during the act of sex. You know the one; wild abandon followed by frantic clutching at the chest. Someone says, "*You okay?*" and then it's lights out.

In general that scenario is less likely than movies suggest but most people are sexual. Not many people get married with the idea of having a non-sexual relationship. Sex is exciting and physical; there is physical arousal and for most people an increase in various metabolic functions. There are non-sexual periods in most marriages. In yours, it might coincide with illness or recovery. Don't be too embarrassed to ask your medical provider for some parameters.

Make sure you both know what is okay (likely everything) and if there are any questions, go ahead and ask your health care provide the embarrassing questions.

Would vigorous sex put undue strain on my heart?

Am I able to take medication for erectile dysfunction?

Will it harm me to have pressure on my chest?

Generally speaking sex is a healthy activity for mind, spirit and body. It can be quite intense or low key and sensuous. In most cases common sense will rule the day. If you are worried, try to distinguish between informed concern and needless anxiety. Most medical facilities will address sex in post-surgical guidelines.

One of the funniest things I ever saw was a graphic on this topic after my last major surgery. It displayed the number of stairs you should be able to climb before having sex again. The funny part was the choice to show some poor guy standing at the bottom of the stairs looking upset while a woman in a negligee stood at the top.

You are married with a child with CHD

Couples marry, typically with the intention of having a fun and sexual marriage and healthy children raised to be healthy adults. When a child is born with a challenge of any kind a number of unanticipated things come into play.

That child will require more time and attention than other children

Parents need to grieve the healthy child they expected

Parents have to decide if siblings of the CHD child need more attention and support.

Parents will have to acquire the knowledge and skills necessary to navigate the medical system.

Parents will need to have exceptional teamwork skills.

Parents will have to figure out a way to ensure that fun, friendship and intimacy do not vanish from their lives.

Parents need to ensure they use external supports to maximum advantage.

These are daunting challenges and not every marriage survives. For one thing all this is tiring and tired couples are not happy couples. As stress mounts they can become angry and blaming, withdraw or delve into unhealthy activities, such as extramarital affairs or substance abuse.

Jim watched with frustration as Tanya's nightly glass of wine turned into two or three and then into a bottle each night. He understood that she needed to "check out" from time to time but not like this. Their lives had been dominated by hospitals and crises for five years. He was not sure that he could live like this anymore.

Valentina had to be at the hospital by nine for her son's appointment. Juan wasn't going to show – again. She didn't know whether he considered his job more important than hers or just found the whole routine too painful.

Aside from trying to manage their own emotions and those of their CHD child they may have to manage emotional issues in their other children.

Cecilia started to have screaming tantrums every time she went shopping with her mother, Beth. Beth wanted them to have some special time that wasn't dominated by her son's needs but this felt like torture. She felt like screaming right back at her daughter.

Emotional management is something of an art form whereby the imperative of experiencing normal emotions is offset by the need to remain composed under difficult circumstances. Generally, "losing it" with loved ones just escalates tension and hurt. Explicit attention needs to be paid to downtime, closeness, recreation and humour. This isn't easy but it reminds people that life is about more than sickness.

Grieving is a term used by many therapists to cover life changing unforeseen losses in addition to bereavement. If your child has CHD, then he/she was never completely healthy but you don't have the imagined perfect child. This can seem selfish to many and they may feel guilt over this particular emotion.

She is wonderful and I love her so much. Why do I look over at healthy children with such envy? I shouldn't feel this way.

However, you do feel this way and those feelings need to be acknowledged and even expressed in a safe place. None of us are perfect loving parents and the appearance of dark or resentful emotions is normal. You also need to allow your spouse to have their moments of doubt. Be the safe place where your partner can go on a bad day.

Likewise you will have to allow each other times where you can't give quite as much.

Bruce was exhausted but wanted Kelly to go on her girl's weekend. If it meant recharging her battery and connecting with her supports he could suck it up for two days.

The therapist in me hates seeing a good marriage break up due to stress. I don't like to see tired hurting people turn on each other. Much is known about marriage and how to make it better. Yes, it is hard and there is often a wall of resentment to overcome, but marriage courses, counselling and shared retreats can help to create a safe space where communication can be improved. My favorite book on the topic of marriage is *Seven Principles for Making Marriage Work* by John Gottman (*see resources*).

A sense of humour helps everything to go better. Every couple has a library of resentments and horrible things perpetrated by the other spouse. If you go searching through that library you will certainly find something to fuel your anger. Your spouse is human and as screwed up as everyone else. Marriages survive because partners learn to bite their tongue before they say something incendiary and see ridiculous where someone else sees drama.

Grief and Loss

> *Grief is the price we pay for love.*
> Queen Elizabeth II

> *There is a sacredness in tears. They are not the mark of weakness, but of power. They speak more eloquently than ten thousand tongues. They are the messengers of overwhelming grief, of deep contrition, and of unspeakable love.*
> Washington Irving

Do you know what a snap band is? It is a therapist trick for addressing intrusive thoughts. You put an elastic band around your wrist and when the intrusive thought comes you snap yourself. I have used a snap band three times in the last three years; on each day my grandson had surgery. The intrusive thought was always:

What if he dies?

After the successful conclusion of the surgery I took off the elastic, went somewhere by myself and sobbed my heart out.

Sometimes the worst does happen and a son, daughter, husband, wife, brother, grandchild is lost. It is our worst fear. But as much as we fear this and desperately as we wish it will not happen, we are better prepared than we think.

I hesitate to state this but one of the most straightforward issues to address in therapy is grief. It is painful and wrenching, but human beings are wired to manage loss.

Our minds and unconscious minds will do most of what is needed to manage grief. There are some important things to understand about grief:

1. It is a significant and dynamic psychological event. Everyone experiences grief in their own unique way but it is to a great extent predictable.

2. Grief can be slowed but it cannot be rushed. It can be slowed by denial, addictive activities or interpreting it as some kind of mental aberration. Grief typically takes much longer than people anticipate. Historically, grief has been seen as taking up to five years for a particularly painful loss (death of a young person, violent death or suicide). Do not let people rush you ("Get over it!") and do not rush yourself.

3. Grieving people go on to live their lives – fulfilling lives – with a missing piece. The person who is lost will never be replaced but over time will take their place as a sad and cherished memory.

4. Grief is weird. People who grieve go through an intensely emotional experience that can have strange manifestations. People who feel the presence of a loved one, or converse with photographs may feel like they are losing their mind but they are simply allowing their brain and spirit to work through the loss.

5. Grief is physical. Somatic symptoms are common during grieving; people will go through periods of fatigue and other physical manifestations of their emotional state.

So what of children and teens who are grieving? There is some good information out there on children and grief but there are some common sense things that work in accordance with their experience and developmental state.

Understanding of death is something that evolves throughout the developmental life cycle. Young children will not understand the implications of death, particularly its permanence. Older children and teens will have a better understanding but may not feel equipped to manage the strong emotions. No matter the developmental stage, all people grieve. As I mentioned before, the ability to grieve is strongly wired into the human psyche.

Children of all ages respond best to honesty tempered to their cognitive ability and level of maturity. Direct and honest information will help them in their own process. Depending on the age, emotions may emerge in play or drawings. Allow children the opportunity to express emotion in their own way. Do not push them to talk or find the words for what they feel.

They will continue to require the normal structure, routine and discipline with allowances for the circumstances. Unless they are very young, their participation in mourning rituals (visitation, funerals) is desirable, but don't force them into a situation where they are too frightened or overwhelmed.

Children who love a parent or sibling often have a profound sense of abandonment and require reassurance that they will continue to be loved and cared for. This may seem obvious to you but a fear of abandonment runs deep in children. Your reassurance that, despite this terrible pain, life will continue is important. They will be reality testing for a time, wondering when the next disaster is going to occur.

Manage but don't hide your own emotions. You are sad and overwhelmed and you need to use your supports and engage those who can help hold you up. Seeing an emotional parent can be scary for kids but in the end it is part of being human. Seeing an upset parent won't hurt children but emotional abandonment might. You and hopefully your larger family and social circle will have to be there for them.

Achievement and risk

*Living at risk is jumping off the cliff and
building your wings on the way down.*
Ray Bradbury

We need risk in life; and we need risk to achieve. Without it we stagnate and sit around. Maybe we lose ourselves in unhealthy or addictive activities. While parents everywhere are protective of their kids, it is a major preoccupation of parents of CHD kids. Often, if we believe that we can't do something we won't.

When you venture into new territory or try to achieve something difficult, you might fail, hurt yourself or feel stupid. It takes a degree of self-esteem and even arrogance to do things that fall outside your comfort zone. Risk can be fun.

I have always liked climbing and have no fear of heights. In another iteration, I might have been a mountain climber. A few years back I reluctantly decided not to take the Grouse grind in Vancouver; which is a path up to the top of Grouse Mountain. I knew I would not make it to the top. However, a few years before that after looking at Sioux Mountain across the lake in Sioux Lookout for years, I hopped in my boat, went over and climbed the rock face to the top. Sioux Mountain isn't exactly Everest but for me that was an opportunity to try something new just to see if I could succeed.

On other levels I have been the first training co-ordinator of an aboriginal child welfare agency in Ontario, the first social worker in Ontario to develop a serious clinical response to workplace mobbing and a unique hypnosis approach for Trichotillomania (an impulse control disorder where people compulsively pull out hair).

I owe much of this to the challenges I continually put in my way. And I owe that to the need to transcend the flaws in my physique. This is a gift CHD has given me.

But this is me. Some CHD people will have it better than me and some much worse. I was strongly encouraged by my parents who always worried but never stopped me from engaging the world. What this challenge will be for you or your child I don't know, but it will be necessary for a fulfilling life.

It feels unfair. Living with CHD is challenge enough without the world asking more of us. But accepting these challenges and fully engaging in life will make all the difference.

Resources

Bourne, Edmund J. **The Anxiety and Phobia Workbook**, Newharbinger publications Inc., 2005

Burns, Dr. David D. **Feeling Good: The New Mood Therapy**, HarperCollins Publishers, 1980

Burns, Dr. David D. **When Panic Attacks: The New, Drug Free Anxiety Therapy That Can Change Your Life**, Random House, 2007

The above books are excellent and straightforward resources. Many but not all books on mood use a CBT basis but if my book gets you started then these books will help you further down the path.

Branch, Rhena, Willson, Rob, **CBT for Dummies**, John Wiley and Sons, 2013

Like most "Dummies" books, clear, professional and well presented. My clients are quite tickled when I recommend this and they find out how good it is.

De Shazer, Steve, **More than Miracles: The State of the Art of Solution-focused Therapy**. Binghamton, NY: Haworth Press, 2005

Again De Shazer challenges conventional wisdom in therapy.

Duncan, Barry L., Miller, Scott D., Wampold, Bruce E., Hubble, Mark A., **The Heart and Soul of Change: Delivery of What Works in Therapy**, The American Psychological Association, 2010

To truly understand what works in therapy these guys are the best.

Gottman, John, Silver, Nan **Seven Principles for making marriage work** Three Rivers Press 1999

There are many good books on marriage but Gottman, researcher and clinician, has written one of the best. He is also an engaging speaker with videos available on YouTube.

Lambert, Michael J (editor). **Bergin and Garfield's Handbook of Psychotherapy and Behavior Change** (fifth edition), John Wiley & Sons, 2004

Not a book for a day at the beach but if you really want to know what works in therapy and have an academic bent this is a great source.

Mate, Gabor, **When the Body Says No: Exploring the Stress-Disease Connection**, John Wiley and Sons, 2011

Our body is the repository of our emotional experience. Mate, a physician and writer, articulates this link better than anyone I know.

Heart & Stroke Foundation, **Heart and Soul: your Guide to Living with Congenital Heart Disease** www.heartandstroke.ca

Terrific and comprehensive guide. Straightforward and easy to follow; it covers both emotional and medical issues.

On the web…

http://www.clevelandclinic.org/lp/congenital-heart-disease

The Cleveland Clinic website has a handbook available on CHD

CHD Online Handbook

http://execpc.com/~markc/congenit.html

Congenital Heart Information Network

www.tchin.org

Heart and Stroke Foundation of Canada

www.heartandstroke.ca

Variety Children's Heart Centre, Winnipeg

http://www.vchc.ca

Royal Children's Hospital, Melbourne, Australia

http://www.rch.org.au

Cincinnati Children's Hospital

www.cincinnatichildrens.org

Children's Heart Network, British Columbia

www.childrensheartnetwork.org

Want to look up something on Doctor Internet? These are reliable sources of information. There are many websites on CHD; some consumer driven and some that focus on the medical end. If you are looking for serious information go to legitimate sources; typically Hospitals, Universities, National, State and Provincial government health departments provide excellent information. Avoid "medical conspiracy" sites, and sites frequented by hypochondriacs and the disgruntled.

Padesky, Christine A. Greenberger, Dennis **Mind over Mood: Change How You Feel by Changing the Way You Think** Guilford Publications, March 15, 1995

This a classic Cognitive therapy workbook that is every bit as helpful today as it was when first published twenty years ago.

Pearson, Patricia, **A Brief History of Anxiety (Yours and Mine),** 2008, Vintage Canada

Patricia Pearson's honest, funny and informative account of anxiety is a great personal memoir in the hands of a skilled writer.

Ruiz, Don Miguel; **The Four Agreements, A Practical Guide to Personal Freedom**, Amber-Allen Publishing, 2008

Ruiz loses a few people in the first chapter when he talks about Toltec wisdom but hang in, this is one book I want all my clients to read.

Shorter, Edward How **Everyone Became Depressed: The Rise and Fall of the Nervous Breakdown** Oxford University Press; 1 edition (February 1, 2013)

This book is academic and historical in tone but it has some fascinating things to say about our perception of mental and emotional struggles.

Acknowledgements

I sometimes joke with my daughter Elisa that the best inspiration for my grandson, Griffin will be the old man on the couch in the living room with a beer in his hand watching the Toronto Blue Jays game. But I didn't reach this blissful state by myself. Throughout my life I have been hugely supported.

First I want to thank my mother, late father and sister for lifelong support, love, and when I needed it, challenge. You did everything right.

Thanks to my wife Nina who also manages to set the right tone between support, challenge and expectation.

My daughter Elisa inspires me with the strength and wisdom she brings to supporting Griffin.

Griffin you are just six as I write this but you are bundle of amazing energy and courage.

To my granddaughter, Anna; you are wise and wonderful beyond your years and the best possible sister for Griffin.

Thanks to my son Paul who provides muscle around the house when Dad isn't feeling strong.

Thanks to my clients who are my teachers in life.

And a shout out to a gang of guys who have played golf on the second Saturday of September every year since 1974. When I was a kid we played sports every day. I couldn't keep up. It didn't matter. You never left me out.

Thank you to the excellent team of medical professionals who watch over me in Toronto. I started at the Hospital for Sick Children and moved over to the University Health Network at Toronto General where I have been followed and supported with compassion and professionalism at the Adult

Congenital Heart Clinic and the Pacemaker/Defibrillator Clinic. You bear much credit for any contributions I have made to the world. Many blessings to you all.

Also thanks to the family physicians who have kept the rest of my body working over the years: Theresa O'Driscoll, Robert Minty, and David Marcassa.

Yeah, I have a therapist. She's great, there when I need her, and does BodyTalk too. I have no idea how *that* works but it does for me. Thank you Julia Laidlaw!

Finally, thanks to my watchful editor Claire LeSage. If there are mistakes in grammar or style in this book it probably means I ignored her advice.

The Author

Richard Schwindt is a social worker in Kingston, Ontario where he has a practice in psychotherapy and hypnotherapy with special focus on recovery for targets of workplace mobbing. He is a graduate of Glendon College and the Carleton University School of Social Work, a member of the Ontario College of Social Workers and Social Service Workers, the Ontario Association of Social Workers and the Canadian Society for Clinical Hypnosis (Ontario Division). Richard has worked in Toronto, Sioux Lookout and Kingston, Ontario in a variety of clinical setting for children and adults.

He is author of **Emotional Recovery from Workplace Mobbing**, **The Emotional Recovery from Workplace Mobbing Workbook**, **Emotional Recovery from an Affair**, **Emotional Recovery from Situational Anxiety**, **Emotional Recovery from Marital Separation**, **The Death in Sioux Lookout Trilogy**, **Dreams and Sioux Nights**, and **The Love Duology**.

He has been married thirty-eight years, has two adult children and two grandchildren. His website is www.richardschwindt.ca

Emotional Recovery from Congenital Heart Disease won the Outstanding Book Award (non-fiction) in the 2016 Independent Author Network Book of the Year Awards.

Made in the USA
Middletown, DE
24 July 2023

35677355R00066